A Guide to Psychiatric Examination

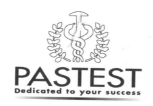

PASTEST
Dedicated to your success

To our mothers, Josephine Aquilina and Pamela Warner

A Guide to Psychiatric Examination

Carmelo Aquilina

MD MRCPsych

Consultant in Old Age Psychiatry
South London & Maudsley NHS Trust
Croydon

James Warner

MD MRCP MRCPsych

Senior Lecturer in Old Age Psychiatry
Imperial College London
Honorary Consultant in Old Age Psychiatry
Central North West London Mental Health Trust

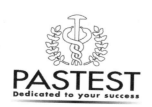

PASTEST
Dedicated to your success

First published 2004

ISBN: 1 904627 14 5

A catalogue record for this book is available from the British Library.

PasTest Revision Books and Intensive Courses
PasTest has been established in the field of postgraduate medical education since
1972, providing revision books and intensive study courses for doctors preparing for
their professional examinations.

Books and courses are available for the following specialties:
MRCP Parts 1 and 2, MRCPCH Parts 1 and 2, MRCGP, MRCPsych, MRCS, MRCOG
Parts 1 and 2, DRCOG, DCH, FRCA, PLAB Parts 1 and 2

For further details contact:
PasTest, Freepost, Knutsford, Cheshire WA16 7BR
Tel: 01565 752000 Fax: 01565 650264
www.pastest.co.uk   enquiries@pastest.co.uk

Text prepared by Carnegie Book Production, Lancaster
Printed and bound by Page bros, Norwich

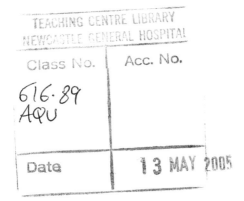

Contents

Foreword

'What did you see me do?' I asked my trainee, at the end of a difficult psychiatric interview. 'Oh, you asked a few questions and just listened, I suppose.' It was a simplistic description of a complex process and I was both affronted and flattered; the simpler it may have seemed to be, the more experience had gone into it.

All of us will have witnessed, or experienced, many kinds of interview - the journalist and politician scoring points; police interrogating the accused; an appointments panel digging beneath the applicant's veneer of confidence; the bland street checklist; an intimate fireside chat; the confessional. And we will all have watched, aghast, as an incompetent clinician approaches a patient with elements of all of these, and wonders why neither of them got anything positive from the process.

The psychiatric examination is complex indeed, and requires the utmost skill. It may be the patient's first contact with the helping services; it will colour the memory of it forever. It may be the first time that the patient has entrusted his life-story to another; it is a privilege that must be accepted with the respect it deserves. It is the psychiatrist's equivalent of the laying on of hands, at once diagnostic, reassuring and therapeutic. And it entails a complicated set of balances.

The interviewer must have a framework in her head of what she wants to achieve, and yet retain the flexibility to approach it from whatever direction is needed. The interview must be open and facilitative, encouraging the patient to take things further and further, like ripples on a pond; but it must have a shape to it, in time and depth, that enables the patient to leave it in reasonable order. A level of distress may be inevitable; psychiatric problems are painful and we can no more avoid it than the pain of physical illness. But that distress must be handled with care. The interviewer must exercise an element of control and yet leave the patient feeling empowered. Wary though they may be of each other, both will need to trust.

All of this takes us back to that finest of balances, between asking questions and listening, and these are equally active processes. Indeed, 'just listening' is perhaps the most difficult bit of all - listening with your ears, to what the patient says, listening with your eyes, to how he says it; listening to your own feelings, to what they may tell you about the patient's distress. Listening to the here-and-now, and to the layers of history that may be crucial to its understanding.

Yes, this is a complicated process and the authors offer a superb guide to its implementation for trainees at all levels, across all disciplines, in both general and specific circumstances, with different age groups and different diagnostic categories. But the book is much more. Anyone reading this forward could be forgiven for giving up in the face of it all. The authors, however, approach the reader with exactly the same combination of firmness and facilitation that they would wish the reader to approach the patient. Psychiatric interviewing is an art-form, but it is an art that can be taught.

Far from being abashed, I closed this book feeling more confident to put my skills into practice. It helped re-awaken in me the conviction that brought me into psychiatry in the first place – that human contact between doctor and patient, difficult though it may be, is the stuff of what we do. Thank you.

Mike Shooter,

President, Royal College of Psychiatrists, 2004

Introduction

This book is intended primarily for medical students and psychiatrists starting their training. It is designed to make life easier during your initial psychiatric attachments, during the first few months of work on a psychiatric unit and when revising interviewing skills before an examination. Other professionals, especially nurses, psychologists, occupational therapists and general practioners may also find this book useful for developing their skills in assessing people with mental health problems. This book concentrates on developing good interviewing skills in a psychiatric setting, but is not a psychiatric textbook. We recommend that it is used in conjunction with a standard textbook to enable you to develop interviewing skills and knowledge of psychiatric disorders simultaneously.

The first two editions of this handbook were published as *The Psychiatric Examination Handbook* in 1996 and 2002 under the auspices of the Royal Free Hospital and Imperial College respectively. We would like to thank Janssen-Cilag Ltd for making their production possible. Since the first edition of this booklet was published we have received many comments and useful feedback from its readers, especially our own students and trainees. Other professionals including general practitioners, social workers and nurses have also found it useful and we hope that this will continue to be the case. Please send your feedback and suggestions to us at PasTest.

Carmelo Aquilina
James Warner

Acknowledgements

In addition to invaluable feedback from many of our students, we would like to thank the following people for advice and suggestions when writing this and earlier editions of this text: Joe Herzberg, Adrian Galea and Mike King. We would like to thank Walter Buscuttil for help with the chapter on post traumatic stress disorder.

We would also like to thank the following for granting permission to use material in this book:

- John F Morgan for allowing us to use the SCOFF questionnaire
- The journal of Clinical Psychiatry for granting permission to use the Appendix to 'The Modified Mini-mental state (3MS) examination'
- and the WHO for use of AUDIT (alcohol use disorders identification test).

Contributors

Dinesh Bhugra Ma, MSc, MPhil, MBBS, FRCPsych, PhD

Professor of Mental Health and Cultural Diversity
Institute of Psychiatry
London

Julia Gledhill MSc, MRCPsych

Clinical Research Fellow (supported by a Wellcome Trust Research
Training Fellowship)
The Academic Unit of Child and Adolescent Psychiatry
Imperial College
London

Sally-Ann Cooper BSc, MBBS, MD, FRCPsych

Section of Psychological Medicine
Division of Community Based Sciences
University of Glasgow
Glasgow

SECTION A

The Basics

1   Why interview?

The ability to talk to and observe patients has always been a fundamental skill of any good healer. Such skill has been overshadowed in most branches of medicine by pressure of time and the advent of medical technology, although it remains fundamental to the assessment of people with mental illness. The psychiatric interview as described in this book is not only crucial for clarifying the diagnosis, but it also shapes the relationship between the mental health professionals and the patient. This in turn strengthens the therapeutic process.

Aims of the interview

An interview is not just an exercise in information gathering, but may have several additional aims. You need to be clear in your mind what you want to achieve in each interview, so that you will tailor your interview to fulfil that objective. The aims of the interview may be to achieve any or all of the following:

1   obtain information about the patient's symptoms and/or problems
2   elicit relevant details of past and present circumstances
3   examine their present mental state
4   clarify the diagnosis of the patient's illness
5   plan or revise management of the case
6   establish a rapport with the patient that allows you to work together to solve the patient's problems and alleviate their distress
7   to be therapeutic in itself; many patients find the simple act of talking through their problems with a sympathetic and attentive listener helpful.

You should be flexible about your aims. For example, if you are asking about past circumstances and this proves distressing to your patient, try switching from a diagnostic aim to one that is supportive and therapeutic.

2   The basic skills

A good psychiatric interview is a dialogue. It is neither a passive listening exercise nor an interrogation, but has elements of both listening and questioning, the balance of which changes according to the dynamic of the interview and the circumstances. For example, after a suicide attempt the patient needs to be allowed time to express their feelings, but the interviewer also needs to know the circumstances of the event and the patient's attitude towards the future. The approach adopted is unique and ever changing according to the interview setting, the patient, the interviewer, and the interaction between them.

A good interviewer will:

1   be non-judgemental in attitude and approach

2   be interested in the patient and their concerns

3   listen to what the patient is saying and how they are saying it

4   observe the patient's appearance and behaviour

5   be focused on the aims of the interview but also flexible during the process of the interview, and will change its focus and style according to what the patient says and how they look

6   be in control of the interview and be able to at appropriate times

   • allow spontaneity from the patient

   • encourage the discussion of difficult topics or feelings

   • stop the patient going into unnecessary detail or wandering off the point.

7   be sensitive to their own and the patient's feelings by being aware of:

   • how the patient makes them feel and what effect they have on the patient.

Techniques used

Most of the significant information that is obtained from an interview is often offered spontaneously by the patient, and a good interviewer is able to establish the right environment for this to occur. However, the interviewer also needs to keep the focus of the interview on the aims of the assessment within the time available. The techniques described below are useful for achieving this.

Questions

This is the most fundamental way to obtain information if it is not volunteered. If you do not ask any questions your patient will feel uncomfortable and confused. If you ask too many questions you run the risk of reducing your dialogue to an interrogation. It is not just the number of questions but also the type of question that is crucial. You need to be aware of the following three types of questioning.

1 **Open question**. This allows the patient to answer the question in their own way (eg 'How is your sleep?'). This is the best sort of question to ask initially, it gives the most reliable answers and allows the patient to feel listened to and appreciated. However, it can produce irrelevant or rambling answers.

2 **Closed question**. This can usually be answered as 'yes' or 'no' (eg 'Do you have any sleep problems?') This type of question is useful if time is short, if non-leading open questions do not work, or to clarify information you get after an initial open question.

3 **Leading question**. This makes it seem that that the questioner is expecting a certain answer (eg 'You sleep well, don't you?'). This type of question may be justified when you feel a patient is holding something back from you (eg saying they are all right but appearing tearful or angry). Use this technique sparingly, if at all, as it can appear aggressive, and may prompt the patient to tell you what he or she thinks you want to hear!

Statements

Statements are used to punctuate a dialogue for a variety of reasons, which are discussed below. You should not set out to use a particular type of statement, but it is important to be aware of the kind of statements you tend to use. You will be able to do this if you are observing someone else or watching a video of yourself. You need to be aware of the following types of statement.

1 **Informative statement**. This is a bland statement of fact (eg how long the interview will last or what the interview is about).

2 **Empathic statement**. This lets the patient know that you acknowledge how they are feeling (eg 'I know this is difficult for you to remember'). Be careful not to use this type of statement too much or in a manner that is patronising or insensitive.

3 **Summarising statement**. This is a recapitulation of what has been said (eg 'So you started to feel depressed after you were made redundant'). This type of statement can be used several times in the course of the interview when you want to check with the patient what you have understood so far. It gives the patient the opportunity to confirm, clarify or refute what you have said. It also demonstrates to them that you have been listening to them, and it helps you be confident about what the patient has said.

4 **Clarifying statement**. This is an admission that you have not understood something and want to know more, eg 'I'm not sure I understand what you mean by "depressed".' It is important not to take certain words at face value as the patient may interpret the term 'paranoid' quite differently to the way in which psychiatrists understand that term. This may also be an invitation to expand on a patient's particular word, phrase or sentence.

5 **Commenting statement**. This is a statement about non-verbal aspects of the interview (eg 'You seemed very upset when you told me about your neighbour'). This type of statement highlights aspects of the interview that require further comments or explanation by the patient.

6 **Self-relevant statement**. This encourages the patient to reveal aspects of him- or herself in response to careful statements by the interviewer about similar feelings, situations, or opinions that they share (eg 'I've been upset myself when I fail at things'). This type of statement makes the interviewer seem more approachable. Be careful not to reveal highly personal information, or be inappropriately friendly. Only use self-relevant statements sparingly, if at all, especially with new patients.

Control

You will need to be able to control the rate, flow and direction of the interview especially during examinations or in busy clinics. The time available is limited and you need to know the reasons why you want to talk to the patient (eg to obtain a diagnosis, to find out how they feel, to help them feel better, etc). The interview needs to be managed sensitively to allow the patient to feel they have been listened to and the interviewer to achieve the aims with which they set out at the start of the conversation.

1 **Silences**. Short silences maintained by the interviewer allow the patient to continue speaking, whereas long silences can make the patient anxious. However, some people will need longer pauses if they are obviously distressed, confused, or slowed up by mental illness. If the person remains silent you may need to move the interview on.

2 **Verbal facilitation**. This can include noises such as 'umm' and 'aha' or 'I see' or repeating (but not mimicking) the last word or phrase the patient has said. This is particularly useful if you want the patient to expand on a topic. It is sometimes misused when the interviewer has no idea how to proceed and keeps using verbal facilitation. Excessive use of this technique can become very irritating for the patient.

3 **Non-verbal facilitation**. This is body language that tells the patient to keep on talking (eg nodding, smiles, waves of the hand, etc). Leaning slightly forward towards the patient is another sign of interest. However, too much eye contact may be threatening or may appear over-familiar. It is important to avoid giving off non-verbal signs of disapproval if the patient makes you feel angry, disgusted, etc. Subtle non-verbal cues can also be used to help interrupt over-talkative patients.

4 **Encouraging statements**. These are used if the patient is reluctant to speak, and in cases where an initial general question and a suitable pause elicit either no answer at all or one that is too brief or vague. Different types of encouraging statement include the following:

- **examples** (eg 'I once had a patient who only felt this way in crowded places'). You may really know such a patient, but sometimes these useful statements are not true. They may be a safe way to introduce a sensitive topic.

- **guesses** (eg 'It almost seems as if you hate your father'). Be tentative rather than dogmatic. If you have guessed correctly and have said the unspeakable the patient may be encouraged to follow it up.

- **motives** (eg 'Are you embarrassed to talk about this?'). Establishing fears or motives will allow you to reassure the patient, clarify your motives and show that you are non-judgemental. Such statements should be made sensitively as they can sound quite challenging.

5 **Discouraging statements**. If time is short and the patient will not stop, gives too much detail or wanders onto irrelevant topics, it is necessary to re-establish control of the interview. These techniques are easier if you set a time limit to your interview beforehand (see below). They include the following:

- **mind the gap** – jump in when there are natural pauses in the conversation
- **interruptions** – interrupt tactfully (eg 'I'm sorry to stop you but I need to move you on to other things')
- **no time for that now** – 'We don't have time to go into all the details now … but we can discuss this point later if there is time'. Only say the second bit of the statement if you really do intend to go back and re-interview the patient later.

Asking sensitive questions

During the interview, sometimes problems arise that are because of the topic rather than the technique. The patient may be reluctant to talk about a topic and the interviewer may be too embarrassed to ask about it. Common topics that cause problems for the novice interviewer are discussed below. Common sense should dictate when to address potentially difficult themes. It may be prudent or practical in some situations to leave these questions for a later interview. If the reason for asking the question is clear to both parties and the subject is introduced tactfully there should be no problem in asking once you have gained the patient's trust. Sensitive topics usually include:

1 **Suicide**. This is one of the few topics about which questions must not be delayed for later interviews. You must ask your patient screening questions as it is dangerous to miss suicidal ideas. Asking about suicide will not increase the risk of it happening. If the patient is suicidal they will often welcome the chance to express their feelings. A good way of starting is to ask 'Have there been times when you thought that you would rather not carry on'. If this question elicits a response you can continue with 'Have you ever made any plans to harm yourself?' and then ask 'What would you do?'. Suicide assessment is covered in more detail on page 67.

2 **Sexual orientation and experiences**. It is often the interviewer's attitude to this subject which makes the topic sensitive. When asking questions about sexual matters it is important not to appear embarrassed, titillated, or disapproving. If you think the patient will be shocked or feel uncomfortable, ask a general question such as 'do you mind if I ask you a few personal questions?' Then it may help both you and the patient to be direct (eg 'At what age did you first have sex?', 'Do you have a partner at the moment?', 'How is the physical side of your relationship?').

3 **Sexual abuse**. This is often a secret and is always a painful subject, so use your discretion when asking about it. It is especially important to ask about sexual abuse in cases of eating disorders, unstable (borderline) personality disorders and self-mutilation. One approach is to ask 'Have you ever had a sexual experience you didn't want?' If you are interviewing children, these questions should be more gentle and non-leading. One approach is to ask the child if anyone has ever touched them in ways that made them uncomfortable or unhappy.

4 **Forensic history**. Your patient probably has considerable difficulty disclosing this, so it is especially important to emphasise confidentiality with regard to this topic. A good way to break the ice is to ask 'Have you ever done anything which could have got you into trouble with the police?' Ask for details of any actual arrests, charges and imprisonments as well as situations where the person could have faced charges if they had been found out. The exception to maintaining confidentiality is when the patient discloses a serious past, present, or potential future crime, such as serious violence towards other people, or sexual abuse of minors. Unless you have warned the patient beforehand, speak to a senior colleague about whether or not to breach confidentiality. If necessary, seek the advice of the General Medical Council, medical defence organisation, or other relevant professional body.

5 **Current and future risk of violence** (see page 100). This situation is difficult for the interviewer because they fear provoking the violence they are asking about and they do not know when violence may occur. Asking about the possibility of violence needs gentle, unhurried questioning, a calm neutral approach and alertness for non-verbal cues of impending violence. A safe setting is essential. If the patient seems angry or aroused simply comment on it (eg 'You seem angry'). If they elaborate, this may allow expression of their feelings without physical violence. Ask them if they consider that the violence is getting out of control or if they intend to do anything about it. If they express hostile feelings towards other people, ask how far they might take those feelings and/or how and in what circumstances they might act on them. If the patient is severely depressed (and especially if they are suicidal and/or deluded), you should ask if they feel that death might be better for other people as well.

3   Developing the skills

The skills required of a good interviewer can only be developed through observation, practice and feedback from colleagues and a supervisor. The psychiatric examination will initially seem rather daunting, but the more patients you interview and see being interviewed the better you will get. The following are some suggestions to help you to learn the skills outlined above.

1   Use a basic psychiatric textbook. Read up or revise the basic features of the major psychiatric illnesses, ideally before you start questioning. At this stage you do not need an advanced textbook but you will need a foundation of basic facts to build upon.

2   Write down a series of headings before you start the interview, and fill in the spaces beneath the headings as you conduct the interview. This has two advantages (especially in an exam or a busy clinic):

   • you will be able to include all of the different parts of the history under the correct heading without having to rewrite it

   • at the end of the interview, any heading for which no information has been filled in will alert you to the fact that you have forgotten to ask about it.

3   It may be better for you (and kinder to the patient) if you initially split your interviews into two or three stages. As your skills and experience increase, you will find you will take much less time to complete the interview.

4   It is perfectly acceptable to glance at checklists to remind you of what signs to look for and symptoms to ask about. With experience you will remember them but in the beginning you will need a little help.

5 It is also helpful initially to look at the diagnostic criteria for the psychiatric condition you suspect. This will allow you to be more confident and consistent in your diagnoses and once you have made enough diagnoses you will remember the criteria easily.

6 After you have assessed your patient, check your assessment with the case notes. This will give you an idea of what you have picked up, or missed! You might be pleased to find that your assessment is better than the one in the case notes or that you have revealed crucial new information (see notes on consent and confidentiality on page 21).

7 After you have seen a case, read up about the psychiatric condition you suspect. There is nothing like having a case fresh in your mind for learning about a diagnosis and retaining that information.

8 Learn with colleagues; ask colleagues to observe you during an interview. You will need the patient's consent to the observer being present and both of you will be bound by the normal rules of confidentiality. This applies even if your colleagues are observing you from the other side of a one-way mirror. You may want to conduct the first few interviews in pairs.

9 Present cases to each other. You will learn how to present cases effectively and confidently. You may pick up better presentation skills from listening to colleagues, or even recognise some bad presentation techniques in yourself.

10 Make use of audio or video recording facilities. If your teaching facility has them see or listen to videos or tapes of experienced practitioners at work. A little later, if you get the chance, video or tape your interview then watch or listen to it with a colleague and/or an experienced clinician. Analyse your questions by seeing what techniques you are using and whether they work or not. Provided you stick to these guidelines such recordings are a very useful way of learning and improving your technique. If you plan to use video or audio recordings you or your training organisation

must keep in mind the guidance issued by the General Medical Council (*Making and using visual and audio recordings of patients*. General Medical Council, 2002 www.gmc-uk.org). This includes obtaining consent, ensuring the interests and well-being of the person takes precedence over other considerations and explicit arrangements for storing and availability of the recording.

11 Try to see as many different people as possible. It is essential to interview patients with a variety of diagnoses which should include:

- depression
- psychosis
- someone who has tried to commit suicide
- dementia
- anxiety
- alcohol dependence.

12 Try to see people presenting in as many different settings as possible. You should not restrict yourself to seeing people presenting to one particular setting. Broaden your experience by seeing people in:

- in-patient wards (psychiatric and medical)
- out-patient settings (including general practitioner [GP] clinics)
- at the patient's home
- in special settings (eg Accident and Emergency units, memory clinics, eating disorder units).

SECTION B

The Psychiatric Interview

4   Preparing for the interview

The initial diagnostic psychiatric interview is the cornerstone of psychiatry. People usually get the most detailed assessment during their initial interview and colleagues who review the case often refer back to this. The initial assessment will also shape the relationship between patient and professional as well as influence the management and treatment plan for the patient. If your initial interview is therefore for someone new to the service it is important to get the best start possible. The interview framework suggested below assumes that this is the initial clinical diagnostic interview. Other types of interview will have different aims and may not necessarily need all the detail mentioned. However, the advice regarding the preparation for and the structure of the interview will still apply.

A good preparation before the interview will pay you back by improving the efficiency and safety of your assessment. In real life not all the preparations may be in place (eg you really cannot rearrange a room if interviewing in your patient's house).The more things you can prepare beforehand the better.

Make sure you are ready

1 **Review all existing information**. If you are seeing a new case as the result of a referral think about the reason for referral (ie who thinks there is a problem, why, why now and what could be going wrong?). This will allow you to start focusing questions once the interview starts. If you are seeing someone already known to services, review other sources of information such as old notes, GPs records etc so you can put the interview into context. Keep an open mind and do not ask questions which simply confirm your initial hunch. Remember established patients can present with new problems.

2 **Have your headings ready**. If you are using pre-written psychiatric headings on your notepaper or a checklist, make sure they are at hand.

3 **Record any demographic information**. It is important to record basic details of the patient's name, age, ethnic origin, marital status, employment status and current housing situation in all cases. If these are not available they should be covered in the initial questions. Demographic data also help focus your assessment and have a bearing on possible diagnosis and management.

4 **Think of things to keep with you**. A packet of tissues is handy in case the patient is tearful.

5 **If there is a risk of aggression, make yourself less vulnerable**. If there is a past history of aggression, or the initial information suggests it, be prepared. Do not interview people alone. Take off your tie, glasses or necklace. Tie back long hair. Prepare the room properly (see below and page 100).

Make sure your interview area is ready

1 **Ensure privacy**. Interviews should always be conducted in private and you should make sure that no-one overhears your discussion.

2 **Ensure facilities are present**. If you plan to perform a physical examination make sure that the right equipment is present (eg stethoscope, ophthalmoscope, sphygmomanometer, tendon hammer, etc).

3 **Arrange the furniture if necessary**. If you are using an interview room with a desk, avoid interviewing across the desk because it puts physical and psychological distance between you and your patient. The chairs should be comfortable, equal in height and arranged at a slight angle to each other if possible so that you can still keep eye contact with your patient but not force it. Your chair should be positioned so you are able to write down notes without having to turn away from your patient.

4 **Make sure the interview setting is safe**. Patients with mental illness are rarely aggressive. However, you should ensure that you are between the patient and the exit, and that the

exit is unlocked. Scan for items that may become weapons. Try to make sure that there is some way of getting help if necessary. Many interview rooms are now equipped with alarm systems; familiarise yourself with the location and operation of this. Ensure that a member of staff knows where you are. If you are interviewing someone who has a history of aggression, it may be better to be accompanied by a suitable colleague.

5 The psychiatric history

The stages of any psychiatric interview for whatever reason and in whatever setting are as follows:

1 introduce yourself and any other people present to the patient

2 inform the patient why you are going to interview them and what is involved

3 seek the patient's consent

4 ask the questions needed and observe the patient to get the information required

5 summarise what has been said to check with the patient if this is correct and complete

6 conclude the interview by reviewing what the aims of the interview were, whether they have been achieved and what happens next.

Remember that, unless you are in an examination or a similar time-pressured situation, if the patient is tired, unco-operative or upset, be prepared to stop your interview and review the case on another day.

Introduction

1 Greet the patient verbally. Introduce yourself and what you do, offer to shake hands if appropriate. Introduce any other people present.

2 Sit down and give non-verbal cues of interest and friendliness.

Orientation

You need to seek explicit consent for the interview and document that you have done this. Broadly, for someone to consent to an interview, they need to:

1 have the capacity to make the decision (ie understand and retain information about the interview and be able to weigh this in the balance)

2 be given sufficient information on what the interview is about so they can reach a decision

3 make a decision without coercion.

To do this you will need to:

1 Explain the **purpose of the interview** and how much time is available. Always underestimate this by at least 5–10% of the available time to allow time for clarifications and recapitulations at the end (see page 59).

2 Explain what you want the **focus of the interview** to be (eg the current problems, response to treatment, etc).

3 Explain the **need to take notes** and to interrupt to allow coverage of essential points within the allotted time span. Some individuals prefer to take notes as the interview progresses, others feel note-taking impedes the development of rapport and prefer to leave it to the end. To begin with you will probably need to take at least some notes; it is unlikely you will be able to remember everything to write down at the end.

4 If you need to **speak to an informant** ask the patient if they mind you speaking to the person in question.

5 Reassure the patient about **confidentiality**. Patients should be informed about who will have access to the notes you make and who will be sent letters relating to your assessment. Remember patients have a right of access to their medical notes. Medical students will report to their supervisor or consultant and the patient must be made aware of this. If speaking to an informant you may want to say that you simply want to ask them questions but not divulge what the patient themself is saying. If the interview is in connection with a medical report or some legal process explain who else will see the report, the information to be given and the reasons for divulging it. If a patient is unable to provide valid informed consent because

of lack of capacity, you may be able to continue with an interview under the common law doctrine of necessity.

6 **Ask if the patient is satisfied**, and reassure or reply as needed, document the above steps and then move on to the main part of the interview.

Taking the psychiatric history

Although we have presented the following headings in what we feel to be a logical order, some authors have different ideas about the precise ordering. The most important thing is that you are able to elicit a comprehensive and accurate history, rather than worry too much about the order in which the information is recorded. Once you are familiar with a particular sequence of headings stick to these and it is unlikely you will miss any out.

Demographic data

If these have not been recorded before the interview (see above) start by asking and recording the patient's name, age, marital, employment and housing status, whether they are detained under the Mental Health Act and if relevant their perceived ethnic origin and religion (if practised).

Ask about the presenting complaints

Start the proper interview with an open-ended general question (eg 'What problems brought you here?') Allow the patient to discuss freely the reasons they feel they are having the assessment. List each presenting complaint with a brief comment in the patient's own words. eg 'feeling low for the last 2 months', 'hearing voices', etc. If the patient has been referred by someone else and the problem has not been mentioned, refer to what the referee wants to know and ask for the patient's opinion about this (eg 'your doctor was worried about your tearfulness – is that a fair concern?'). Allow at least 10% of your interview time for such 'free' talk as it is potentially the most revealing part of your interview. The emphasis here is on breadth of complaints rather than description in depth.

History of presenting complaints

Explore each complaint or concern in turn.

- when did the problem start or if this is unclear, ask when was the patient last well

- did any event precede the problem (eg bereavement, starting a difficult job or course, break up of a relationship, etc)

- how did it develop (time-span, symptoms)

- are there any associated symptoms (ie if a patient reports feeling depressed, elicit other psychic symptoms (eg anhedonia, poor concentration, feelings of guilt, hopelessness, suicidal ideation) and physical symptoms (eg disturbed sleep, loss of appetite, diurnal mood variation etc))

- what effect does the problem have on day-to-day life and compare this to previous functioning (if a patient is not sure what you mean ask them to describe a typical day and whether this is different from before)

- has the patient sought any help and have any of these measures proved effective (include details of any recent or current drug or psychological treatments for the problem).

Attempt to relate the different complaints. For example, if someone presents with symptoms of depression, anxiety and derogatory auditory hallucinations, you should be able to elicit a timeline and details for each phenomenon. Failure to explore each presenting symptom fully is a very common mistake among students and trainees.

Screen for any other problems that the patient may not volunteer, by asking brief questions, this is especially true when no clear idea of the problem is obtained from the presenting complaint or the patient is not forthcoming. All patients should be screened for the following symptoms:

- low mood
- changes in energy

- delusional or obsessional thoughts
- unusual perceptions
- other unusual experiences
- suicidality
- changes in social contact
- sleep problems
- anxiety.

Always be prepared to **re-visit history-taking**, as **other symptoms** may emerge (especially psychotic symptoms) at later stages of the history-taking exercise. An opportunity is given at the end of the interview to ask the patient if there is anything else they think the examiner should know and it is not unusual for new symptoms to be volunteered then.

Ask an **informant**, if present, separately if possible what has been their view of the problem, any opinion on what caused it and any concerns they have about the effects on the patient or themselves.

Past psychiatric history

'Have you had any mental health problems or seen a psychiatrist in the past?'

This section should be a record of similar or any other psychiatric symptoms in the past.

1 Include instances when problems were not treated, or were treated by the GP. For example previous episodes of depression may have gone unrecognised by doctors, but may be evident from the patient's description.

2 Record previous contacts with psychiatrists and details of hospitalisations. In particular, the length of hospitalisation (or detentions under the mental health act) can provide a clue to the severity of illness. In individuals with a very complex past psychiatric history, it may not be possible to document all previous admissions. At least attempt to record the number of admissions, when they first began and details of the last three or four.

3 Specifically ask about any past diagnoses, attempts at deliberate self harm, and treatments (this includes psychological treatments and counselling as well as drugs, depot medication and courses of electroconvulsive therapy (ECT)).

4 Ask about the state of health and level of functioning between episodes. It is important to identify whether the patient returns to work/social functioning between periods of illness.

In someone who has been continuously ill since their first presentation, the distinction between the history of presenting complaint and past psychiatric history becomes blurred. Under these circumstances, for relatively short illnesses (say up to six months) it may be advisable to treat the whole history under 'history of presenting complaint'. For longer illnesses, you will require some judgement about where in time to place the watershed between history of presenting complaint and past psychiatric history.

Past medical history

'Do you have any current serious illness: Have you had any major illnesses, accidents or operations?'

'What medicines are you taking?'

'What is your physical health like at the moment?'

List major physical illnesses and treatments in chronological order and any current prescribed or self-prescribed drug treatment. Screen for specific morbidity such as head injuries, epilepsy, heart disease, strokes, diabetes, hypertension, jaundice (eg as a result of hepatitis) and any allergies to prescribed drugs. Screen for current physical symptomatology (eg breathlessness, constipation, dizziness, etc).

Family history

'Can I ask you about your family?'

Information on the following relatives should be routinely elicited:

- parents or people who raised the patient
- siblings
- children
- other significant relatives. You may find it easier to record family details in diagrammatic form (called a genogram) as shown below.

For each relative ask: about age (or when and at what age they died), employment, social circumstances, major health problems (or cause of death), history of psychiatric disorder, alcohol and drug misuse and the quality of the relationship with the patient.

Ask if there were long periods of separation from the parents, how did or do the family get on with each other.

Any major psychiatric illness in more distant relatives is also important.

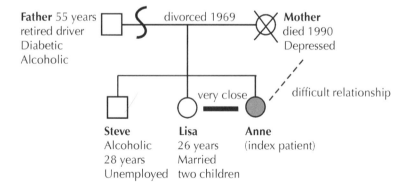

Father 55 years
retired driver
Diabetic
Alcoholic

divorced 1969

Mother
died 1990
Depressed

difficult relationship

very close

Steve
Alcoholic
28 years
Unemployed

Lisa
26 years
Married
two children

Anne
(index patient)

Personal history

'I'd like to know a bit more about you. Can I ask you questions about your past?'

One of the ways you can understand a person better is to know how they came to be who they are. A life history can be very lengthy and detailed as a glance at published biographies will show. Fortunately you do not have to record life stories in that depth. To keep things relevant and brief, use standard headings. These should prompt non-leading, closed questions to help you cover the necessary facts. You may need to explore relevant episodes in some depth (eg death of a child or parent) and skim over others (eg each house move). Try to include the following:

Childhood

- area where they were born and raised
- any known problems around birth (time spent on Special-Care units, prematurity)
- delays in developmental milestones (eg delays in walking and/or talking)
- what are childhood memories of the family like, eg family atmosphere (including major upsets such as deaths, divorce of parents), separation from family (eg for prolonged hospitalisations), relationship with siblings.

School

- details of primary and secondary schooling, school leaving age
- truancy or school refusal, bullying
- relationships with teachers and peers
- exams taken and qualifications
- further education (university, professional, etc).

Occupations

List chronologically each job, duration of employment and reasons for leaving. Also note any periods of unemployment.

Relationships

- current relationship – if married or cohabiting, when it started, quality of relationship
- past relationships – how long they lasted, how and why they ended (ie separation, divorce, death)
- if in a relationship and there are no children is the patient trying to have children? (Or if elderly why did the patient have no children?).

Sexual history (see page 10)

- age at menarche/puberty
- first sexual experience (both masturbation and with another person)
- any instance of sexual abuse
- current or past sexual difficulties (eg any difficulties including loss of libido, impotence, delayed ejaculation, or vaginismus).

Habits and dependencies

'Do you smoke, drink alcohol, or take any drugs which the doctor has not prescribed?'

Record any use of tobacco, alcohol, solvents and any prescribed or illicit drugs. Note whether their use is regular or not, if it is regular consider pattern of use, any withdrawal symptoms, and physical, psychological and social impact. See page 102 for details of taking an alcohol history and page 106 for details of assessing drug dependency.

Forensic history

'Have you done anything which could have got you in trouble with the police?'

Record all offences, whether convicted or not (and mentally ill people tend not to get charged or convicted). Make special note of violent crimes, sexual crimes and persistent offending (see page 10).

Present social situation

'I'd like to ask you about how and where you now live.'

Many patients with mental health problems experience high levels of deprivation and social exclusion. You should attempt to identify details of their current social circumstances.

Housing

- type of housing: whether single or communal, rented or owned
- state of house: eg no heating, dangerous stairs, not accessible to wheelchairs, etc
- proximity to amenities like shops and public transport
- other members of the household, and their relationship to the patient.

Social support

- friends, relatives
- neighbours
- voluntary and statutory organisations
- daily activities:
  - Ask the patient to describe a typical day.
  - Ask about social activities such as church or social clubs.
  - Identify problems with daily activities such as shopping, cooking, laundry and cleaning.
  - Do they drive?

Finances

- do they manage their own finances? If not, who does?
- do they have any debts or financial worries?
- what benefits are they currently receiving?

Personality

`How would people who know you describe you?'*

Personality traits are an individual's coping strategies for every aspect of their life. They are formed in adolescence and shape behaviour and thinking throughout life. Although personalities are unique, certain broad traits seem to crop up in people (eg obsessional characteristics). Personality traits are common but specific personality disorders are relatively uncommon. You should therefore refer to traits rather than disorders unless you are sure of your diagnosis and the criteria used to make that diagnosis. Be aware that the effects of illness can give a misleading impression of personality, eg hypomanic people will appear confident, depressed people will withdraw from social contact, etc).

Assessing personality can be quite difficult in an initial interview. No individual can objectively describe their own personality so an account from an informant is important. If you have to assess personality only from the patient, eg during an exam, you must state that this is the patient's own self-description. The emphasis should be on consistent patterns of behaviour throughout life.

The following are some of the clinically useful areas to explore:

1 *Attitudes to others* – ie friendly, keeps friends, trusting?

2 *Attitudes to self* – ie likes self, confident?

3 *Predominant mood (affect)* – ie cheerful, optimistic?

4 *Leisure activities and interests* – ie hobbies, activities undertaken for fun (eg TV, radio, newspaper)?

5 *Reaction pattern to stress* – ie able to cope with stress well, what is the coping strategy?

More common (and more easily recognised) personality traits are:

1 **Obsessional**. These tend to be perfectionists, conscientious, rigid and can be preoccupied with rules, lists and procedures. It can be adaptive in certain professions (eg academics) but becomes maladaptive when it causes distress to themselves and others. People with this trait are

more prone to get depressed when life events ruin their routine.

2 **Paranoid**. These patients have lots of ideas of reference, are sensitive to even implied slights, have over-valued ideation regarding their rights, and are quarrelsome. They fall out with people, rarely make friends and can become socially isolated.

3 **Schizoid**. These personalities tend to be interested in mechanical matters or objects and not very interested in people and social relationships. They can be eccentric, aloof and rude or abrupt with other people. They rarely develop relations with other people unless they have the same interests and then the relationship is not deep.

4 **Inadequate**. These personalities have life-long dependency on others. They usually pair up with a more dominant personality and can function well while this relationship lasts. They usually present to psychiatric services when their partner dies, they divorce, etc and they cannot cope with decisions or take the initiative.

5 **Antisocial**. These personalities show an inability to empathise and see the effect of their actions on other people. They can be superficially charming but ultimately callous, self-serving and aggressive. They have poor, fickle and inconsistent relationships. They are more likely to commit crimes, abuse children or spouses, take drugs or abuse alcohol. They seem to be very good at manipulating other people including professionals.

Read any psychiatric textbook for more details of these and other personality disorders.

6 The Mental State Examination (MSE)

The assessment of mental state (MSE) is the part of the psychiatric examination which students find most difficult to present. The problem in our experience is that students are very observant but are not familiar with either the headings or the vocabulary to describe their observations. Most of the MSE can be carried out in parallel with history-taking: appearance and behaviour, affect, speech can all be readily observed and commented upon without having to ask any questions.

A source of confusion here is distinguishing which information is recorded under 'history' and which under 'mental state'. The MSE should be restricted to information about the current episode of illness, and observations during the interview. Try to avoid 'normal' or other bland, unhelpful terms and instead describe what is there. What is normal to you may not be what is normal to other observers. Another clinician should be able to identify the patient you present purely on the basis of your description of the mental state.

The following headings and sequence are conventional. They should be used when recording or presenting a case. This will make life easier for yourself and for the people you are presenting to or who are reading your records. Refer only to positive findings in your presentation unless absence of a particular symptom is relevant (eg where it might be important in making a diagnosis of schizophrenia).

Appearance and behaviour

The aim here is to paint a 'pen-picture' of the patient, using a repertoire of standard adjectives. From your description, the person to whom you are presenting should be able to identify your patient. The difference between appearance and behaviour is analogous to that between a photograph and a film. Your observations and description should include the following headings:

Appearance

1 **Level of consciousness**. This may range from drowsy to aroused.

2 **General impression**. This may include body build (eg slim, athletic), an appearance of physical illness (see page 58), posture, cleanliness, evidence of weight loss, any evidence of self-harm etc.

3 **Face**. Eye contact, expression (eg glum, frightened, angry, disdainful, etc), or appearance being blank and expressionless (eg in Parkinson's disease or severe depression) should all be noted.

4 **Dress**. This may be bizarre, dirty, revealing, inappropriate to the weather. Extra layers of clothes or loose clothing may indicate anorexia or covered up arms and legs may be a sign of intravenous drug abuse.

Behaviour

1 **Motor**:

- speed – ie fast movements (eg agitation, restless legs (akathisia), dystonic movements), or slow movements (eg retardation in depression, Parkinson's disease, drowsiness)

- repetitive or rhythmic writhing (choreoatheosis), chewing of mouth or trembling lips in tardive dyskinesia

- odd movements – eg grimacing, echopraxia (mimicking examiner's movements) rituals (in obsessive–compulsive disorder (OCD) see page 88), tics or other stereotyped movements.

2 **Attitude to examination**. Patients may be friendly, hostile, suspicious. Note 'catastrophic reactions' of anger and irritability in cognitively impaired people when their memory is probed informally during interview or during formal memory testing.

Speech (see also thought disorders)

A common problem for beginners is deciding what to put in this section and what to put in the section on thought form (see page 45). It may be simpler to use the speech section to record abnormalities of the mechanics (or form) of speech. In general, if there is a problem in the way the thoughts are reported through speech, then it may be better to record these abnormalities under disorders of thought form. The distinction is arbitrary and there is a large amount of overlap with the section on thought form. Do not worry too much about which bit of the mental state you record your findings in as long as you pick up the problems. If the patient says anything significant or bizarre then record appropriate examples of what the patient has said whenever possible. Properties of speech to note down include the following.

Production

1 **Spontaneity** – usually in depression, impaired level of consciousness, or a preoccupation with psychotic phenomena, the patient only speaks in response to questions and usually the volume is low and speed is slow.

2 **Speed** (pressured or retarded) – pressure of speech can be found in hypomania and slowed down speech (retarded) can be found in depression, with the latter there is also poverty of content and low volume.

3 **Loudness** – patients speak in a low voice when depressed and at high volume when hypomanic (or angry!).

4 **Quantity** – do they say too much (eg hypomania) or too little (eg depression).

5 **Quality** – is there any dysarthria (ie is production of words impaired)?

Form (see also page 45)

1 **Neologisms** (new words invented by the patient), verbal stereotypies (or stock words or phrases; existing words or phrases used inappropriately) and circumlocutions (vague phrases used instead of words, eg the 'whatsits') are found in schizophrenia or dementia.

2 **Punning (a play on words)** and clang associations (links between sentences resulting from similar sounding words), are both to be found in hypomania or frontal lobe dysfunction.

3 **Expressive dysphasia** (Broca's or non-fluent dysphasia) comprises broken sentences with normal words but no following of grammar or sequence. This is found in neurological disorders such as stroke or dementia.

Content (see also page 40)

1 **Obscene words** may be used by people who are angry, intoxicated, in delirium or frightened. They can also be found in Tourette syndrome (where it is called coprolalia).

2 **Poor fluency** – you should note if the patient is not easily able to express what they want. This can be the result of:

- *poor education or shyness* – you can understand what they are trying to say but they cannot say it well

- *thought disorder or circumstantiality* – where even you cannot understand what the patient is trying to say

- *receptive dysphasia* – (Wernicke's or fluent dysphasia): words are appropriate and sentences are formed but the sentences do not make sense because the patient does not understand what is being said to them and by them. This is difficult to distinguish from word salad (or drivelling, see page 46)

- *echolalia* – the patient repeats what is said to him – this is rare but can occur in schizophrenia

- *perseveration* (inability to shift topic in response to a change in questions), is found in concrete thinking (see page 47 below), a form of schizophrenic thought disorder, and also in frontal lobe dysfunction.

Mood and affect

Another common difficulty even among experienced clinicians is the difference between the mood and affect. Readers may find it easier to use the following distinction. Affect is an observable manifestation of emotion, eg sadness, joy, disgust. Affect is only observed by others and can change frequently and rapidly. Mood is a longer-lasting and less changeable emotion which is less prone to internal or external stimuli. Predominant mood is best evaluated longitudinally by questioning the patient. Affect is not always in keeping with mood (eg you can appear happy for short periods even when you are feeling generally low).

When recording the mental state, you should record subjective (ie the patient's assessment) and objective (your assessment) of their mood. This could be normal (euthymic), elevated (elated) or depressed. You should also note the predominant affect and stability of affect as described below. Especially during a short interview, objective mood and affect may be regarded as synonymous.

Affect

You should observe the patient throughout the interview to note predominant affect and changes of affect. Affect can be described under any of the following headings.

1 **Type of affect** – anxious, sad, happy, angry, disgusted, ashamed, detached.

2 **Intensity** – mild or intense emotion.

3 **Stability** – either in degree of intensity, eg blunted or labile, or in variability of type, eg changeable or restricted:

- *Blunted (flat)* – this is when the normal variability of range of affect (reaction to either good or bad news does not occur or occurs in a limited way). This may be caused by mental illnesses such as schizophrenia or depression and by physical illnesses such as Parkinson's disease or hypothyroidism.

- *Labile* – this is when affect changes quickly from one extreme to the other in a very short time, often in reaction to other minor events (eg whilst crying at the loss of a relative they may suddenly laugh at the sight of someone). Lability may occur with dementia and conditions affecting the frontal lobe, during extreme stress, hypomania, drunkenness and mixed affective states.

4 **Appropriateness** – whether the observed emotion is appropriate to the situation or not. Inappropriate affect is to be found in conversion disorder (the 'belle indifference' of hysteria), after severe trauma or emotion, intoxication, the mask-like expression with antipsychotic drugs, frontal dementia and hebephrenic schizophrenia.

5 **Congruity** – whether or not other observations tally with the observed affect (eg patient has low mood but very relaxed body posture). Incongruent mood occurs when the reaction to some event is the opposite of what is expected, eg laughing when bad news is given. Before deciding that the affect is abnormal it is necessary to check what the patient thinks as sometimes people laugh to avoid showing the expected emotion, or the person's opinion on the event is at odds with what is expected (eg they may be pleased that a relative has died). Incongruent affect occurs in schizophrenia, antisocial personality traits and hypomania.

Mixed affective states can occur where there are simultaneous signs and symptoms of both elation and depression (eg crying whilst singing).

Mood

The general questions to ask are 'how have you been feeling lately?' or 'can you describe your mood?' and ask the patient to describe how they have been feeling in the weeks or months prior to the interview. Mood can be described under any of the following headings.

1 **Type of mood**. Common mood states include:

- *Depression* (see page 71). This may be associated with psychomotor retardation (being slowed up) or agitation. The patient will usually complain of feeling low (depressed) or lacking in enjoyment (anhedonia) or energy (anergia). Try to elicit feelings of guilt, worthlessness and hopelessness. Screen for biological features such as diurnal variation of mood, disturbed sleep, change of appetite or weight, loss of libido etc.

- *Hypomania and mania* (see page 74). This is often manifested by elation (objective and subjective elevation of mood), irritability, expansiveness, grandiosity and over-activity. Ask about excessive spending, risk-taking, sleep (often reduced) and energy levels (often excessive). You may see pressure of speech or flight of ideas.

- *Irritability*. Patients can become irritable simply by being in hospital or asked questions. Abnormally irritable moods last longer and are often reported by informants or by the person who refers the patient. You may notice the patient being loud, critical easily annoyed, uncooperative, tense, and restless. This is an easy mood to pick out in the interview room and care must be taken if the patient becomes violent (see page 100).

- *Anxiety* (see also page 85). The patient can look frightened, startles easily, fidgets with clothing, and there may be physical signs of anxiety, such as tremor, dry mouth, difficulty with concentration, etc. (See also Appendix 4 on page 160 for information on physical conditions which may cause anxiety). Remember that anxiety can occur with depression in agitated depression.

- *Alexithymia* is the inability to feel or describe any sort of mood. This can occur in chronic schizophrenia, after strokes, and in chronic post-traumatic stress disorder (PTSD) states.
- The term *euthymic* is used when mood seems to be normal.

2 **Intensity** (eg mild, moderate, or severe). One way to examine intensity is to ask the patient to rate their mood on a scale of 1 to 10 (eg 1 being the worst they have ever felt to 10 being the best). Delusions and/or a significant disruption of functioning are also indicators of severity.

3 **Chronicity**. Is the problem with mood relatively recent (weeks or months) or longer lasting (years)?

4 **Stability**. Is the problem changeable or not over time (eg mood changes from depressed to euphoric over time) or in response to external events (eg low mood worsens or starts in response to an unhappy event).

An uncommon alteration of mood is **delusional mood**. This is not usually related to affective disorder. The patient feels anxious and uneasy and feels that there has been a change or that something is about to happen – a feeling that 'something is in the air' but they do not know what. It is a primary delusion in schizophrenia and may precede autochthonous delusion. The patient thinks that the new delusional idea was the reason they had been feeling that way.

Thought

Thought is usually assessed through the content of speech and to a lesser extent behaviour. Thought is assessed in two ways – the form the thought takes and the content of the thoughts themselves.

Abnormal thought content (also known as beliefs)

As these are usually mentioned in the presenting complaint there is no need to repeat them in detail in this section of the history. However, in this section you should record examples of abnormal thought content that the patient is experiencing or recounting at the time of the interview.

Patients will usually respond well to anyone taking an interest in what they have to say. The examiner needs to keep a professional distance from even the most bizarre or strange beliefs expressed and not directly contradict, challenge, or diminish the importance given to their beliefs by patients. It is just as bad to collude with their beliefs to get them to express their ideas as this cannot be sustained and will lead to the patient losing their trust in you later. It is possible to explore obviously delusional beliefs and probe for further information without agreeing with them. It is best to question the patient with an attitude of sincere interest and to gently probe any inconsistencies or illogicalities.

The two main groups of abnormal beliefs are categorised by whether there are delusions or not.

Delusional abnormal thoughts

Delusions are significant symptoms with important diagnostic and prognostic implications. It is worth learning the definitions of delusions off by heart as it is both clinically useful as well as a common question in examinations.

A delusion is a false belief which is:

1 maintained even despite proof to the contrary
2 out of keeping with the patient's social, cultural and educational background.

Delusions are of great personal importance to patients as they make sense of distressing and confusing experiences, they usually dominate their thinking and actions, and many put the patient at the centre of things.

Delusions are usually held with absolute certainty by the patient. It is never worth trying to reason people out of these beliefs as the normal rational process does not work. Imagine someone trying to argue you out of believing that it is colder at the North Pole than at the Equator. No matter how hard they try, you just would not believe that the Equator was colder. This is the intensity with which delusions are held. Although you should not ridicule or challenge these beliefs you should gently probe how firmly they are held.

Delusions can wax or wane depending on the underlying primary disorder, during which time the patient may doubt whether the delusion is true or not. Although strictly speaking these are not delusions, they are usually called 'fading' or 'emerging' delusions and this is significant in determining co-operation with and response to treatment.

Types of delusions

1 **A primary delusion** arises 'out of the blue' without any identifiable precedent. This can be in the form of a delusional idea (or delusional intuition). The patient may relate the delusional idea to a normal percept (eg a person sees a plane flying overhead and then believes he is the new Messiah), in which case the primary delusion is in the form of a *delusional perception* (a first-rank symptom). There may be a delusional mood (see page 39) or a *delusional memory*. These primary delusions are usually of momentous significance and place the patient in the centre of things.

2 **A secondary delusion** arises out of an underlying mood, from another psychotic phenomenon or from a defect in cognition or perception and is understandable in that context. It arises out of an attempt to integrate (understand) the primary morbid experience. For example a primary delusion of being followed can give rise to secondary delusions of persecution. In the latter case the beliefs emerge slowly and retreat with treatment.

3 **Systematised delusions** are a series of delusions which fit in to an internally consistent system of beliefs, eg hearing voices and feeling they are being poisoned or spoken to from the television might be seen to be part of a plot by the secret services. It is the result of an attempt by the patients to make sense of what is happening to them and the systematised delusions usually follow on from an earlier psychotic experience.

4 **Mood-congruent delusions** can occur in depression or mania. In these cases the beliefs fit in with the prevailing mood. Examples are that a person's internal organs are rotting, that they have lost all their money or that they are being persecuted for something they may have done in the past in depression. In mania a patient may believe they have special powers or huge wealth.

5 In **folie à deux** two people are very close and share a delusion. Usually the two people live isolated from the outside world and the dominant member of the pair has induced the delusion in the passive partner.

Themes of delusions include the following:

1 **Persecution** – the patient believes he is being monitored, followed, harassed, or harmed by a person or group of persons.

2 **Reference** – significance is read into ordinary events eg from news reports, ordinary conversations, or posters. If not held with delusional intensity these are known as ideas of reference.

3 **Control/passivity** – explanations for feeling that thoughts, actions, feelings are being controlled by an outside agency (first-rank symptoms).

4 **Thought possession** – Thoughts can be experienced as being broadcast, inserted, or withdrawn (first rank symptoms).

5 **Jealousy** (Othello syndrome) – the patient thinks their partner is being sexually unfaithful. This is commoner in men with alcohol problems and is associated with a risk of violence.

6 **Amorous** (de Clerembault's syndrome) – patient thinks another person (usually of a higher social status) is secretly in love with him and communicates this in oblique ways. The person involved sometimes bombards their imaged lover with messages, gifts etc. This can lead to stalking or even violence if the love is not reciprocated.

7 **Grandiose** – patient thinks he has a grandiose identity or power. Sometimes they feel that events happening in the world have been caused by them.

8 **Guilt** – patient thinks they are guilty of any minor or imagined misdemeanour or of bad events which happen elsewhere.

9 **Worthlessness** – patient thinks that he is not important to anyone and is in fact a nuisance.

10 **Nihilistic** (Cotard's syndrome) – patient thinks that internal organs have disappeared or rotted away or that family, possessions or even the world has been destroyed or disappeared.

11 **Infestation** (Ekbom's syndrome) – patient thinks that insects or animals are infesting the skin or body.

12 **Misidentification** (Capgras syndrome) – patient thinks other person (or rarely an object) is not the real person (or object) but has been replaced by a close substitute.

13 **Fregoli syndrome** – a single persecutor impersonates several people familiar to the patient. This syndrome is named after a stage magician who was famous for his disguises.

14 **Hypochondriacal** – patient believes that he has an illness despite extensive investigations and no clinical signs.

Non-delusional abnormal thoughts

1 **Overvalued ideas** are strongly held, dominate life (and conversation) but are not always illogical or culturally

inappropriate. They usually occur singly and are not normally associated with other psychopathology. An example is someone preoccupied with the harmful effects of fluoridation of water. You should try to distinguish delusions from overvalued ideas.

2 **Phobias** (see page 85) are exaggerated, irrational and persistent fears (or even frank panic attacks) when exposed to specific stimuli. The fears are felt to be unreasonable by the patient and tend to interfere with normal functioning. Fear, avoidance and panic may even be brought about by a thought rather than actual proximity or contact with the trigger. Types of phobias include:

- **Simple phobias** – these include fear of heights, animals, bridges, flying etc

- **Social phobia** – fear of social situations where the person may fear saying the wrong thing, being looked at, being asked to speak to a group, being the object of other people's scrutiny, eg at parties, meetings, etc

- **Agoraphobia** – fear of open spaces or crowds or buildings with people when there is no obvious way to leave a crowded building. The patient typically avoids the situation (and can become housebound). If they do go out they will only stay in places where there are easy (and unobtrusive) exits or they are accompanied by someone else.

3 **Obsessional symptoms** (see page 88) (eg thoughts) are recurrent, distressing and intrusive and are recognised by the patient as being their own but senseless. These unwanted symptoms are resisted unsuccessfully and both the symptom, and the resistance, cause distress. The obsessive symptom is often followed by a compulsive act like checking, counting, arranging, cleaning, etc.

- **Ruminations** – the obsessive symptom is not a single thought but a series of thoughts round a theme (eg is there a God?).

- **Ideas** – these are distressing ideas which come into one's mind (distinct from primary delusions) (eg one's husband is being unfaithful).

- **Memories** – these are distressing memories which come unbidden into one's mind (eg of not passing an examination); distinguish these from the flashbacks in PTSD (see page 90).

- **Imagery** – these are distressing images (eg of a naked relative); distinguish from hallucinations or pseudo-hallucinations (see page 79).

4 **Suicidal ideation** is part of depression and is dealt with on page 67.

5 **Hyponchondriasis** is where a person fears they are ill in spite of repeated negative findings on medical examinations and tests. This is not a delusion as it is not bizarre or out of keeping with cultural beliefs but can be just as distressing or disabling. The belief is accompanied by repeated attempts to get the doctor to check for the undiagnosed illness and a negative result will only confirm to the patient that the disorder is too small to be detected, the test was wrong or the doctor incompetent. Sometimes hyponchondriasis can border on delusional as the ideas can be bizarre and resist all evidence to the contrary.

6 In **dysmorphophobia** the patient believes that a part of their body is ugly, misshapen or otherwise not right in a cosmetic sense.

7 **Eating disorders** (see page 108) are indicated by disturbance of body image, preoccupation with weight and food and low body weight.

Abnormal thought form
(also known as formal thought disorder)

The form of thought is how thought content is organised to form coherent thoughts and sentences. Abnormal thought form occurs when the patient fails to follow conventional semantic and syntactic rules of language. This is another way of saying that the patient does not follow the usual language constructions and speech is less meaningful as a consequence. Abnormal thought form cannot be generally probed for. You need to spend some time with the patient speaking freely. It is very important to record verbatim examples of thought disorder here. Disordered forms of thinking usually suggest schizophrenia and can manifest as alterations to fluency and flow.

1 **Fluency** – various degrees of loss of coherence and direction of speaking can occur with increasing difficulty in understanding what is being said.

- *Circumstantiality* – an over-detailed, over-inclusive account which finally tells you what you asked but makes you wait and sweat for it! This can be a normal personality trait, a feature of obsessional and pedantic personalities or a manifestation of elevated mood, mild confusion and intoxicated states (including, but not exclusively, alcohol).

- *Loosening of associations* – the connection between ideas is lost with no logical connection followed within paragraphs. Thoughts become vague ('woolly'), oblique and irrelevant to the topic being addressed. The patient never seems to answer the question asked. In extreme cases conversation is incomprehensible and is called drivelling (or word salad). It can be a sign of schizophrenia, hypomania and severe dementia.

2 **Flow** – various types of changes in speed, and deviations or interruptions to the flow of thought can occur:

A *Changes in speed* – pressure and poverty of thought.

B **Interruptions to the flow** –
Thought blocking is the sensation of thoughts suddenly stopping. It is experienced as being caused by an external agency. It may last from seconds to minutes and the patient cannot remember what they had been trying to say. The patient may experience it as thought withdrawal.

This rare phenomenon should be distinguished from fatigue or distraction from whatever cause.

Perseveration describes when the flow of thought gets stuck and does not move on to a different topic. It occurs in organic brain disorders and in schizophrenia and depression.

C **Deviations of the flow**:

- *Derailment* – is similar to thought blocking but the patient is unaware of what has happened and continues on a different topic after a few seconds. This loss of meaningful continuity between words or phrases preserves grammar and syntax. It occurs in schizophrenia.

- *Tangentiality* – is when you do not get an answer to what you asked but can follow the logical sequence of sentences as it veers away from its goal. This is different from derailment where you have an interruption in the grammar and logic of the sentence. It is also different from flight of ideas in that it stays within the general topic. It occurs in schizophrenia and with obsessional personality traits.

- *Flight of ideas* – is when the patient veers away from the goal and deviates much more into other subjects than tangentially. There is usually some connection between successive themes although this may be obscure. This is strongly suggestive of mania and is usually associated with pressure of speech (see above).

3 **Funny words** – These are words used unusually or completely new words invented by the patient. Examples include punning, neologisms (completely new words), clang association (abutting two words with similar sounds) and stock words (normal words given an idiosyncratic meaning).

Although letting the patient speak freely is the best way of eliciting formal thought disorder, one way to test specifically for abnormal thought form is to ask the patient to interpret an abstract concept (eg what is the difference between a dwarf and a child) or explain a proverb (eg what do you mean by 'too many cooks spoil the broth'). Keep in mind that the patients' level of education and cultural background may put them at a disadvantage. Also remember that frontal lobe dysfunction can impair abstract thinking (see page 140)

Abnormal thought form should be distinguished from expressive non-fluent dysphasia (see above) where there is usually no delusional belief and the patient is older and usually has signs of cognitive impairment or strokes.

Perceptions

These are usually hallucinations but there may be other alterations of sensory percepts.

Hallucinations

Hallucinations are perceptions arising within the mind without any external stimulation of sense organs (ears, eyes, touch etc). They are as intrusive as obsessional thoughts but the patient does not recognise them as arising from within themselves. Most hallucinations occur without any obvious external trigger.

Unless someone volunteers the fact, or is clearly hallucinating in front of you, it is imperative that you ask a direct question such as 'Do you ever have unusual experiences, such as hear noises or voices talking when you are on your own?' (see page 77 for further details)

Hallucinations can be classified in a number of different ways.

Modality

1 **Visual** – elementary hallucinations (eg noises or flashes of light without other sensory modalities) are more likely to be organic or alcohol-induced; complex hallucinations (eg seeing a well-defined face or animal) are more difficult to attribute as a true hallucination as they may be distortions of visual precepts (ie illusions).

2 **Auditory** – crude hallucinations (eg noises) are more likely to be organic. Complex hallucinations are more likely to be functional and can take several forms:

- *second person voices* – directly addressing the patient (includes command hallucinations which are voices giving instructions to the patient)

- *third person voices* – two voices arguing about or discussing the patient (first-rank symptom)

- *thought echo* – voices echoing thoughts before or after they happen (first-rank symptom) or the related

- *commentary* – a voice or voices talking about the patient's actions before, during or after they have happened (first-rank symptom).This can give rise to a secondary delusion of someone observing the patient in some bizarre way.

3 **Olfactory** – usually of an unpleasant smell. It can occur in depression (where it may be thought that the patient is unclean or their body is rotting), schizophrenia (where there is a persecutory or bizarre explanation), or organic disorders.

4 **Gustatory** – commonly a feeling that something tastes different and this is interpreted as being the result of poisoning or adulteration.

5 **Tactile** (superficial) and somatic (deep) – the former is the experience of having insects or other things touching the body and the latter is usually felt as organs being touched, electric shocks going through the body and being pregnant. They may occur in schizophrenia but the sensation of insects crawling on the skin is to be found in cocaine-induced states, and alcohol withdrawl.

Complexity

1 **Crude hallucinations** are simple precepts (eg noises, lights) and at the other extreme are complex hallucinations (eg seeing a vivid image of a person). Crude hallucinations are usually caused by organic factors.

2 **Complex hallucinations** are usually the result of functional psychoses, although organic disorders, such as Lewy body dementia, temporal lobe epilepsy and migraine, can cause very complex hallucinations.

Trigger factor

1 **Functional hallucinations** – a normal percept triggers off a hallucination in the same sensory modality (eg hearing the voice of the devil whenever a shower is turned on). The hallucination can carry on when the original trigger has stopped.

2 **Reflex hallucinations** – a normal percept triggers off a hallucination in another sensory modality (eg seeing faces at the bathroom window whenever a shower is turned on).

3 **Hypnogogic or hypnapompic hallucinations** are commonly reported. These are hallucinations occurring when someone is going to sleep or waking up respectively. They are not usually significant.

Other perceptual abnormalities

1 **Illusions** – are misperceptions of actual stimuli and these can be normal or occur as a result of exhaustion, anxiety, drug-induced states, conditions of poor lighting and are very common in delirium.

2 **Pseudo-hallucinations** – are not perceived to be arising from outside the individual and usually lack the same intensity and realism as true hallucinations. The patient has insight into the symptoms but cannot dismiss the imagery. It may be difficult to distinguish true hallucinations from pseudo-hallucinations. Both phenomena may occur together. The

so-called 'widow's hallucination' is a common example where a recently bereaved person sees the dead person but realises that this is not real and accepts that the person is dead.

3 **Depersonalisation and derealisation** describe the feelings of the patient that they themselves have changed (depersonalisation) or their surroundings have changed (derealisation). It is an unpleasant feeling as if the person or the world round him has changed. In derealisation there may be an altered perception of the size of the surroundings or objects (eg the illusion that the room is bigger (macropsia) or smaller (micropsia), people or objects seem to be artificial or mechanical, etc.) The 'as if' phrase distinguishes this mood state from a delusion. This feeling of detachment can be found in normal people when extremely tired or with extreme emotions but is also found in depression, anxiety states, organic syndromes and schizophrenia.

4 **Capgras syndrome** – is an altered perception where a person or object or even area looks the same but has lost the feeling of familiarity which leads the patient to think that they have been changed by an impostor or imitation. This can occur in schizophrenia, depression, or in dementia and other neurological disorders.

5 *Déjà vu* is a feeling of familiarity in a new situation and *jamais vu* not feeling this sensation of familiarity in situations they have already been in. They occur in normal people but can also be a sign of temporal lobe epilepsy.

Cognitive Assessment

Cognition is the global 'sum' of the brain's higher level information-processing functions, such as memory, and lower level functions, such as the sensory system.

This part of the mental state examination can seem daunting to the beginner. It need not be as long as the trainee knows what is being tested, why, and when to do more than just the basic tests. If there is no sign during history-taking of a cognitive problem or people are not at high risk for cognitive impairment then all that is needed are a few basic tests which are described below. More detailed information about testing is given on pages 139 and 161.

The various domains which should be routinely recorded in all patients are:

1 level of consciousness
2 orientation
3 attention and concentration
4 memory: short- and long-term.

Testing while you take the history

Most basic cognitive tests can be performed informally during history-taking. If you introduce yourself to the patient at the beginning of the interview and then ask the patient if they can remember your name after a minute then you have tested their memory (albeit rather crudely). Observe for any drowsiness or reduced level of consciousness. When you are asking about their jobs, children or places where they have lived ask them to list them in a particular order, eg from oldest children to youngest or first job to last. You will then have tested their attention and concentration – though this would be also apparent to you whilst taking the history. Orientation can be tested informally by asking people to confirm their name, age and date of birth, and (if you have prepared for it beforehand by checking the time yourself) how long the interview has taken.

Formal testing

When it comes to formal examination it will help you to introduce cognitive tests in a non-threatening way, eg *'Now I would like to ask you a few questions to test how good your concentration and memory are. These are questions which we have to ask everyone and should not take too long. Are you happy with this?'* Once the patient is happy to proceed then test the following domains in a basic way.

1 Level of consciousness

This can be defined as the degree to which one is able to be aware of one's own self and the environment. It is fundamental to all other cognitive functions – if it is impaired then you cannot really test other domains as they will inevitably be impaired as a consequence. You do not need to formally test it – clinical observation is enough – but tests of orientation, and attention and concentration will confirm your impression. You need only to describe what you have observed, eg 'the patient was yawning, and kept closing his eyes throughout the interview.

2 Orientation

This is the awareness of one's position in self, time and place. This is traditionally divided into orientation to (awareness of) time, place and person but includes accurate awareness of the passage of time. The sequence of loss in orientation (and the sensitivity of the test) occurs in the following order:

time ➜ date ➜ place ➜ person

Disorientation to time and the passage of time is the most sensitive and disorientation to person is the least sensitive. During history-taking you may have noted that the patient may be vague about when they were admitted or how long they have been on a ward. However, be aware that people who are in-patients (especially those in long-term residential care) will be vague about date or time because there are few cues as to what time or day it is.

Age disorientation (asking people how old they are and date of birth), though strictly speaking this is not orientation to person, can be asked at this stage; it is a good way to screen for memory problems, especially in older patients.

- **Orientation to time**.

  'Without looking at your watch, can you tell me what time it is?'

  Record the actual and estimated time. Anything more than an hour out is deemed inaccurate. At the end of the interview you may want to check the time again and ask the patient how long did they think the interview had taken – mild disorientation can be picked up in this way.

- **Orientation to date**.

  Although not necessary, the following sequence of questions is suggested.

  'Can you tell me what year we are in?'

  'Can you tell me what season we are in?'

  'Do you know what the date today is?' (answers should include the day and month)

  'Do you know what day of the week it is?'

  Anyone in care or on wards – especially in the long-term – may be disoriented to time and date. When the month or season has changed in the last week allow some leeway. People will tend to remember dates with emotional links better, so asking people what the date is on their birthday will usually produce an accurate answer even when they have some cognitive impairment. For dates you can accept an answer within two days of the actual date as accurate. If they get the date wrong it would be useful to tell the patient what the date is and then ask them again about a minute later; in this way short-term memory has also been tested.

- **Orientation to place**.

  'Can you tell me where we are now....?'

For hospital assessments you should then proceed as follows:

  '....for example could you tell me the name of this clinic or hospital?' (if this is their first visit they may not know so ask what sort of a building it is, eg a school, church, etc)

  '... what floor are we on?' (this is difficult in multi-storey hospitals so an approximate answer may be acceptable)

  'What town or city is the hospital or clinic in?'

  'What county or state are we in?'

For home assessment proceed as follows:

  '... for example could you tell me your address?' (house number or name, street name, town)

'What town we are in?'

'What county or state we are in?' (if this has not already been given in the address)

- **Orientation to person**.

  Knowing one's own identity and name is the basic level of orientation. It is rarely affected except in severe dementia, dissociative disorders (hysterical amnesia) or delirium. A quick way to test it is to ask people what their name is at the start of the interview (eg *'before starting can I check your name so I can be sure I am interviewing the right person?'*).

3 Attention and concentration

Attention is the ability to focus on a particular stimulus or task. A common example is not paying too much attention to a lecture but focusing attention as soon as the lecturer calls out your name. After the lecturer has drawn your attention to the lecture and has asked you a question then you will continue to keep your attention focused on the question until he picks on someone else. *Concentration* then is the ability to sustain attention for a period of time.

To test attention and concentration in a routine examination a good simple test is Reverse sequence, ie *'Can you tell me the days of the week in reverse order?'* A slightly more difficult variant is the months of the year in reverse sequence. If the patient needs clarification explain they need to start from December (or Sunday) going backwards to January (or Monday). Note if the patient makes any mistakes (and how many) or is particularly slow. Alternative tests are:

1 **Counting backwards**. *'Can you count backwards from 20 to 1?'*

2 **Reverse spelling**. Choose an easy five letter word like 'black' or 'world' and ask them to spell it forwards first. If they make any mistake correct them. Then ask them if they could spell it backwards. This test may not be useful if English is not the patient's first language.

3 **Serial subtraction**. Ask the patient to subtract 3 from 20 and to keep on subtracting 3 from the result until they get to zero. If the patient is having some difficulty start by demonstrating the sequence from 26 to 23 and allow them to carry on from 20. Do not allow the patient to write anything down or use their fingers to subtract. Simply note if the patient makes any mistakes (and how many) or is particularly slow.

4 Memory

There is some controversy and confusion over the descriptions of long-term and short-term memory which are used differently by different authors and different disciplines. We suggest that the following terms and definitions be used.

Short-term memory (also known as immediate recall)

This refers to any information kept in mind for about 30 seconds. Information is kept in the working memory longer by rehearsal (eg mentally repeating facts to ourselves just before an examination) and removed by moving our attention to another thing (ie distraction). It is subject to recency (retaining the most recent facts) and primacy (retaining the initial facts). The maximum number of pieces of information retained in working memory is about seven at one time.

The test of choice is digit span which also depends on attention and concentration but is a better test of immediate memory.

'Can you repeat these numbers after me in the sequence I told you and then backwards. For example if I tell you 1 ... 2 ... 3 ... then you have to say 1, 2, 3 and then 3, 2, 1. Do you understand?'

Start with three random numbers and make sure you say them clearly and loudly with a pause in between numbers. Continue with an increasing sequence of numbers and ask the patient to repeat them in the correct and then reverse order until two successive wrong answers (both forward and backward sequences) are given. It is best to write down the numbers beforehand or as you are saying them because otherwise it becomes a test for your memory as well. A series of random numbers for quick use is printed in the Appendix

2 on page 157. Report the number of correct numbers remembered forward or 'forward span' and backwards or 'reverse span'. A normal adult forward span is 6 ± 1 and a reverse span is 5 ± 1.

Long-term memory (also known as delayed recall)

This is any information which is retained after a few minutes of attending to other tasks. The minimum test you should perform is to ask the patient to repeat a name and address after you, ie *'I am going to ask you to repeat a name and address after me. I want you to listen carefully because after about five minutes I will ask you to remember it for me. Are you ready?'*

Then give an imaginary name and address which you should be familiar with, eg

1 Alan Smith

2 22

3 High Street

4 Brighton

5 East Sussex.

Repeat the name and address up to three times (note how many attempts are needed as this is an indication of ability to learn new information). Ask again approximately five minutes later. Record how many items out of the five are remembered and any confabulation (eg saying the name 'Robin Smith').

Recommended supplementary tests which test other types of long-term memory (so called 'remote' memory) are questions concerning:

1 name of the current Prime Minister

2 any item that has been in the news in the last two weeks.

You may however want to tailor these questions to something you think appropriate to the person you are interviewing because these are subject to the effects of age, education and culture. For example, ask people what year they were married, what year they retired, what years were their children born, when they got their first job, etc. With such personal memories it is impossible to verify their accuracy without an informant.

Insight

Insight is not an all or none phenomenon and there are degrees of insight. Insight is subjective and the reason for assessing this is to see whether the patient and doctor share the same ideas about what is wrong and what to do about it. If they largely agree then co-operation is more likely. Insight should be recorded in the form of the patient's answers to the following questions:

1 Is the patient aware that there is anything wrong?

2 Is the problem within the patient or external?

3 If there is anything wrong, does the patient think it is as a result of an illness?

4 If an illness is it physical or psychological?

5 If psychological, can it be helped?

6 Is the patient willing to accept help (if so, what help will they accept)?

Reaction to the patient *(Rapport)*

At the end of the interview you should ask yourself 'How did the patient make me feel?' This question is important because your feelings towards a patient influence your diagnosis and management. Your emotional reaction to an interview may be a pointer to the diagnosis. For example, patients with mania may make you laugh, depressed patients may make you feel sad, and psychotic patients may make you feel confused. A good rapport can be had with people who are hypomanic. When one feels uneasy or uncomfortable with someone it may suggest schizoid, paranoid, or borderline personality traits. However, do not rely solely on analysing your reactions when making a diagnosis. Be wary of inappropriate feelings towards the patient whether this is attraction, disgust, or hostility. Discuss these feelings with a colleague or your supervisor.

Overview

1 Summarise the patient's account of his problems briefly and ask the patient to confirm, clarify, or refute. This will also make the history clear in your mind.

2 Ask a final question: 'Is there anything else you wish to tell me?' This may reveal unexpected psychiatric complaints or other significant information in their personal history.

3 Explore any relevant symptom or problem the patient might mention.

7 The physical examination

People with mental health problems are just as likely to have physical illnesses as any other person of their age. People with chronic mental health problems are indeed more likely to have physical ill health. In the elderly patient mixed pathology (and iatrogrenic disease) is much more common.

It is therefore good clinical practice for all new patients to have a systems review and physical examination which must include a neurological assessment. If the psychiatric examination is performed for other reasons (eg during an exam or as part of training) then a shorter physical is more practical. In this book we are concentrating only on the physical signs relevant to the psychiatric examination. Please refer to a medical textbook and appendices 3 and 4 for more information on the physical signs and illnesses and their significance.

Region	What to examine	Possible findings and significance
General	Body build (thin or obese)	Chronic psychotropic use causes obesity; myxoedema and Cushing syndrome also cause obesity Thinness occurs in anorexia, depression, self-neglect due to chronic psychosis, chronic ill health, or dementia
	Body asymmetry	Strokes
	Colour	Jaundice in intravenous drug abusers or alcoholics
	Smell	Smell of alcohol or foetor hepaticus in alcoholics Bad smell if poor self-care in depression and chronic psychosis Smell of urine indicates incontinence
	Gait	Shuffling in Parkinson's (drug-induced or otherwise) Difficult in strokes or other neurological problems
	Tremor	Lithium toxicity Parkinson's or drug-induced tremor Hyperthyroidism
	Skin	Lanugo (downy) hair in anorexia Piloerection (chicken-skin appearance) in opiate withdrawal (cold turkey) Sweating in anxiety, drug and alcohol withdrawal Spider naevi in alcoholism
	Movement	Slowed down in Parkinson's, oversedation by drugs, or depression
Face	Shape	Moon-like in Cushing syndrome
	Neck	Neck mass in thyroid disease Carotid bruits indicate risk factors for stroke
	Skin	Scars indicate head injury or self-mutilation
	Nose	Nasal septal defect with cocaine use Red and bulbous nose with alcoholism
	Parotid glands	Enlarged in anorexia and bulimia

continues ...

Teeth		Poor in people with chronic psychosis from self-neglect
		Eroded from inside in bulimia from repeated vomiting
		Broken in people with alcohol problems (through falls or fights)
Eyes	Pupils	Argyll Robertson pupil in neurosyphylis, brain tumour, or intracranial bleed
		Altered pupil size in drug intoxication/withdrawal
	Eyes	Staring and bulging in hyperthyroidism
	Eyebrows	Less prominent in hypothyroidism
	Fundi	Prominent and swollen from raised intracranial pressure from any cause
	Eye movements	Ophthalmoplegia in Wernicke's encephalopathy, a complication of alcohol withdrawal
Hands	Skin	Staining with tobacco
		Palmar erythema from alcohol abuse
		Scarring from self-injury
		Excoriated skin from repeated washing in obsessive compulsive disorder
	Pulse	Fast with anxiety
		Irregular with atrial fibrillation and other arrhythmias (a risk factor for strokes)
	Knuckles	Lacerated or calloused from induced self-vomiting (Russell's sign)
	Tremor	Slow resting tremor in Parkinson's disease/Parkinsonism
		Fine tremor at therapeutic levels of lithium becoming coarse with toxicity
		Coarse tremor in anxiety, withdrawal symptoms
		'Flap' with liver failure in alcoholics

continues ...

Arms	Tone	Cog-wheel rigidity in Parkinson's
	Power and reflexes	Reduced/asymmetrical in strokes
	Skin	Scars from self-harm
		Injection marks and thrombosis from intravenous drug abuse
	Axillary hair	Can be absent in anorexia if started before puberty or alcohol misuse
Chest	Heart sounds	Irregular or murmurs may indicate risk of strokes
	Breasts	May be atrophied in anorexia if it starts after puberty (however, athletic women might have the same findings without having anorexia)
Abdomen	Liver	May be enlarged in alcoholism
	Skin	Striae in Cushing syndrome
		Caput medusae in alcoholism
	Pubic hair	Can be absent in anorexia if started before puberty
Legs	Skin	Pretibial myxoedema in hyperthyroidism
	Tone	Cog-wheeling in Parkinson's
	Power and reflexes	Asymmetrical in strokes
		Reflexes stronger in hyperthyroidism, delayed ankle reflexes in hypothyroidism

8 Ending the interview

1 Come to a conclusion depending on what the purpose of the interview was. For example, say what you think might be wrong with the patient, comment on their progress with treatment, etc.

2 Answer any questions the patient might have.

3 Thank the patient for his/her time and patience.

4 Sign and date any notes you have written.

SECTION C

Interviewing in Specific Situations

9   The suicidal patient

Suicide is an uncommon but devastating consequence of a mental illness – usually, but not always, depression. Being 'suicidal' might mean any stage of the continuum:

hopelessness ➔ suicidal feeling ➔ suicidal wish ➔ suicidal ruminations ➔ suicidal plan ➔ suicidal attempt

Patients do not necessarily have to move through this sequence to become suicidal. The stages shown are merely increasing levels of intent (and therefore risk).

What to look for

Look carefully for non-verbal cues of distress or despair. Also, look for visual signs of self-neglect, alcohol abuse (eg smell), which increases the chances of suicide, and for signs of deliberate self-harm (eg tentative cuts to the wrist).

What to ask

Assessment should be on an individual basis but the sociodemographic risk factors should also be kept in mind when assessing the chances of suicide (eg being male, single, socially isolated and mentally ill is a worrying combination of risk factors).

Recent events must be carefully examined, as must suicidal motivation (which is usually mixed) and background social factors. Assessment should be in a quiet, unhurried setting. Start the interview with a non-directive, open question, allowing ventilation of issues and feelings important to the patient; build up trust and rapport by avoiding a judgemental approach (always be aware of one's own feelings eg exasperation). Try to stay empathic, understanding and keep a position of unconditional positive regard. Where possible obtain a collateral history because someone with active suicidal intent will minimise descriptions of the attempt to gain another chance.

If the person has not attempted suicide

Communication of suicidal intent can be indirect, eg by complaining of hopelessness, or by somatic complaints of depression. However, suicidal ideation can also be expressed directly with anything from vague expressions or more specific threats. Do not be afraid to ask about suicide. It does not increase the risk of suicide and most people feel relieved that they can discuss it. The sequence of questions could be as follows:

1 *'Do you still get pleasure out of life?'*

2 *'Do you feel hopeful from day to day? / Do you think things will turn out well?'*

3 *'Are you able to face each day? / Do you ever wish you would not wake up?'*

4 *'Do you feel life is a burden? / Do you wish it would all end?'*

5 *'Have you ever thought of ending your life?/ At the moment is there anything to live for?'*

6 *'Are you able to resist the thought of suicide?'*

7 *'Have you thought about the method of suicide?'*

8 *'Have you ever tried anything?'*

Occasionally you may want to ask the following questions to assess risk more precisely.

9 *'How likely are you to kill yourself?'* If you have concerns about a person's openly expressed suicidal feelings but cannot make up your mind about the degree of risk this very challenging question could be used with caution. This question picks up situations which are likely to occur or recur (such as marital conflicts or an impending eviction) which would make the person more suicidal.

10 *'Is there anything that might make you feel worse?'*

11 *'What might stop you from trying to kill yourself?'* This question identifies protective factors which might reduce the chances of a suicide attempt, eg strong religious conviction.

If the person has attempted suicide

If you are seeing someone after an actual suicidal intent then the sequence of questions indicated above should be used but look for indicators that the attempt was serious (and therefore at high risk of repetition). These are:

- attempt was premeditated and actively prepared for, eg had bought a rope, collected tablets
- precautions were taken to avoid intervention, eg the attempt was carried out in isolation or timed to minimise risk of discovery
- suicidal intent was communicated prior to attempt
- 'final acts' were carried out in anticipation of death (eg suicide note or will)
- violent, active methods or drugs were used that the patient knows to be lethal
- person believed act would be final and irreversible
- person states aim was to kill himself/herself
- person regrets surviving the attempt
- no actions were taken to get help after the attempt
- numerous previous attempts had been made

After a suicidal attempt it might be useful to use that event as an opening question. Asking the patient to describe the day starting from first thing in the morning gives you a good idea of mood and whether the event was planned or impulsive.

Practical points

1 **If there is no sign of mental illness**. Being suicidal is not necessarily a consequence of mental illness. If you suspect a situation like this then seek the advice of a senior colleague or a specialist.

2 **Openly expressed intent**. This may be an attention-seeking act but it may be very serious. Sometimes people who have decided to kill themselves seem very calm and serene as

they now feel that there is a way out. Elderly people (especially men) do not express these ideas lightly. Explore openly expressed intent as you would when picking up intent through questioning.

3 **Alcohol** is only to be taken as a serious indicator if the person drank to be able to carry out the act or if the person is likely to be intoxicated frequently (ie a similar high-risk situation happens often).

4 **Drug overdose.** If the suicide attempt involved taking drugs then the risk is best gauged by asking about the patient's idea of the drug effect rather than the objective risk. For example patients may think 50 capsules of paracetamol are harmless or that 10 mg diazepam is extremely lethal. If the patient 'cannot remember' then you should ask an informant.

5 **Self-harm.** 'Non-suicidal' deliberate self-harm is common and is usually a 'cry for help', a response to being angry at someone or an attempt to manipulate a situation. There are usually no indicators of serious intent (commonly no attempt is made to conceal the attempt), the self-harm may be trivial (although sometimes the patient causes unintentional serious harm to themselves through accident or lack of knowledge).

6 **Homicide as part of suicide.** Please remember that sometimes suicidal ideation is accompanied by thoughts of harming others (as a way of saving them from the catastrophe the patient thinks is happening or will happen). Keep this in mind when assessing any suicidal patient who has significant relationships (eg spouse or young children).

10 The depressed patient

Low mood is very common; everyone feels sad at times. It is when the low mood is severe and persistent that it is deemed to be clinical depression. Depression has several characteristic symptoms which are present in up to 10% of the community. If depressive symptoms are present but do not meet the criteria for a depressive illness then talk about depressive symptoms. Depressive symptoms must be present for at least two weeks (International Classification of Diseases (ICD-10) diagnostic criteria) for a diagnosis of depression. When talking about depression keep in mind the following adjunctive labels which help convey an idea of the prominent symptoms of the depression.

Agitated depression occurs when motor over-activity is prominent. The converse is retarded depression, in which slowing down of mental and physical activity can reach the level of stupor. Both are descriptive labels.

You can also talk about the presence or absence of biological features, and the presence of psychotic ideas.

What to look for

The patient shows a restricted range of affect but usually appears sad and can be tearful. Some people can be so slowed down that they may appear stuporous or mute (psychomotor retardation). Speech may be slow and quiet. Especially in older people, the predominant motor feature may be agitation rather than motor poverty. Physical signs of anxiety symptoms are often present. There may be signs of self-neglect. Look out for signs of physical ill-health as a result of poor appetite – especially dehydration. Be careful not to miss any signs of attempted self-harm, such as tentative cuts to the wrist.

What to ask

When interviewing someone with depression adopt an unhurried empathic approach. Responses to questions may be delayed as a result of psychomotor retardation. In severely depressed patients, the low mood may colour the whole history content. For example, a patient may look disparagingly on their past history, personality and current relationships. Under these circumstances a collateral history is vital. The interview should investigate the following symptoms of depression:

- sustained low mood or tearfulness (lasting at least two weeks)
- anhedonia (lack of capacity for enjoyment)
- anergia (lack of energy)*
- diurnal variation, usually feeling worse in the morning*
- loss of interest in hobbies etc
- poor concentration or memory
- poor sleep, especially waking up early* (rarely, increased sleep)
- loss of appetite and weight (rarely increased appetite)*
- lowered libido*
- feelings of guilt or worthlessness
- feelings of hopelessness or suicidal ideation
- negative thoughts and ruminations
- delusions which are usually mood-congruent (eg of poverty, guilt, or nihilistic) **
- preoccupation with physical health symptoms (when delusional can be nihilistic).

*these are known as biological features of depression

**features in psychotic depression

Practical points

1 Do not be shy to enquire about **suicidal ideas**. A truly depressed patient is highly likely to have thought about suicide (see page 67). Rarely, depressed patients want to kill their loved ones as a way of taking them out of their imagined desperate situation. Keep this in mind and ask about thoughts of harming other people (see page 11).

2 **Anxiety symptoms** are commonly present so screen for these.

3 **Psychomotor retardation** can present as cognitive impairment (depressive pseudo-dementia). Sometimes it is very difficult to tell the two apart but look out for 'don't know' answers which are commoner in depressed people who do not have the motivation to try even a wrong answer.

4 **Physical ill health** is both a cause and a consequence of depression so thorough physical examination and investigations are needed. This is especially important in older people (see Appendix 3 and chapter 23).

5 People can be unhappy for many reasons but it is the intensity and duration of these unhappy feelings that make it into a clinical depression. Low-intensity but chronic low mood can be called **dysthymia**.

11 The manic patient

Elevated mood is similar to depression in that it is abnormal only when present to an abnormal extent or for an abnormal length of time. Mania is different from hypomania only in degree and is usually defined as when day-to-day functioning is impaired. Normal people can feel euphoric or happy and act accordingly but these periods are usually in response to a happy event, last for a brief period and are not so intense that normal life is disrupted.

What to look for

Manic patients can appear over-active, dress unusually and speak loudly, profusely and without hesitation (pressure of speech), though with a lot of deviation (and flight of ideas). They may be disinhibited in speech and manner. Some may be irritable, eg because their plans are being delayed by some silly fool asking them questions. Irritability is more common than elation in older people. Look for:

- bizarre or dishevelled dress
- elated and/or irritable mood
- over-activity/restlessness and decreased need for sleep
- distractability
- over-familiarity with strangers

What to ask

You should always try to obtain an informant's account as the changes from normal may be subtle and the transition may have taken place over a long time. Interviewing someone with mania can be very difficult. Try to keep the focus of the interview on the patient, avoid answering personal questions and use control techniques to keep your interview on track. Ask for:

- excessive and/or reckless spending
- decreased need for sleep (ask how many hours sleep per night)
- over-ambitious plans for the future (eg in excess of what you expect from the account of the person's previous abilities) with disorganisation and/or several projects initiated at the same time
- grandiose ideas or delusions (of grandiose powers rather than identity)
- disinhibition, over-familiarity, reckless behaviour or increased sexual energy
- flight of ideas
- pressure of speech, possibly with punning.

Enquire about past episodes of high mood and whether or not medication to control this has been stopped by the patient or a doctor.

Practical points

1 Elevated mood can be very difficult to pick up and distinguish from happiness in a normal person if it is subtle and or non-bizarre. An **informant** is important – ask them if this elevated mood had ever occurred before (even if not to the same extent), what the patient's past abilities were and what the effect has been on day-to-day life (including relationships with others, health, work and finances).

2 The patient may have **no insight** whatsoever or may have partial insight, admitting that their mood is elevated but denying that there is a problem and saying that they like feeling this way.

3 The patient will not usually complain of their condition and may resent any suggestion that their mood needs to be brought down. This will lead to some **difficulty in co-operating** with questions and even less co-operation when treatment is mentioned.

4 If the patient is likeable and jolly then **your feelings** towards them might lead you to give them the benefit of the doubt and give them allowances for their behaviour that you might not allow with other patients.

5 If the patient is **over-familiar** this can lead to problems in keeping an appropriate professional boundary so ask a chaperone to come in with you.

6 Remember **stimulant substance misuse** can be a cause (eg amphetamine, cocaine, ecstasy, etc).

7 If **delusions** are present, it may be difficult to distinguish from schizophrenia (see page 77).

8 Some **dementias** (especially frontal lobe dementias) can present in this way, as sometimes can delirium (see page 93).

12 The psychotic patient

Psychotic patients are suffering from prominent and persistent delusions and/or hallucinations and they have limited or no insight. Psychosis can occur in severe depression, mania, schizophrenia, organic states, drug intoxications (especially amphetamine and ecstasy), or other rarer presentations such as erotomania, Capgras syndrome, delusional disorder and paraphrenia. The emphasis in this section is on schizophrenia.

Schizophrenia is a syndrome where delusions (usually bizarre and self-referential), hallucinations (usually auditory), abnormal thought forms or disorders of movement or volition may be present. The syndrome can occur once, intermittently, or it may run a chronic course. It most commonly starts in younger people, and may be triggered by the use of drugs.

What to look for
Delusions

Unless expressed openly, delusions are not directly observed but their effects may be seen. People may be wearing strange clothes or accessories such as aluminium foil over the head to stop thoughts from being inserted. If seeing patients at home, windows may be blocked or doors may have lots of locks. The patient may show you writing which may show persecutory thinking or be difficult to follow. Chronically psychotic patients may be self-neglected or show signs of long-term use of neuroleptic drugs, eg tardive dyskinesia.

Hallucinations

It is uncommon to see someone hallucinating but once seen it is never forgotten. People may be easily distracted by what they are hearing, they may be talking back to the voices or looking frightened, laughing, or becoming irritable for no apparent reason.

What to ask

Delusions

It may sometimes be difficult to elicit abnormal delusions because some patients do not discuss their delusions readily as they are aware that people might think they are mad. However, some sympathetic 'free time' at the beginning of the interview may encourage them to talk. There are several 'probe' questions which you can ask:

- *'Has anything been worrying you lately?'*
- *'What's been on your mind?'*
- *'Has anything odd been happening to you lately that others find difficult to believe?'*
- *'Is there any plot or conspiracy going on?'*

Asking the appropriate prompts to elicit delusions may not be enough. Once delusional beliefs are mentioned or you have information about them from an informant you might be able to ask specific questions about their delusions:

1 Ask what the symptoms mean to the patient, and how they came to that conclusion. The abnormal reasoning behind their beliefs is more important than how bizarre their beliefs are, though the latter are usually a strong clue!

2 Discover how strongly their beliefs are held by asking if there could be (or even offering) alternative reasons or explanations for what they are experiencing.

3 Investigate their insight into their experiences – this is not just the strength of the delusional belief (see page 58).

4 Ask what effect this is having on them and what they intend to do about it.

Once a delusion is out in the open you may be expected to give your opinion or collude with the belief. You should tactfully say things like *'I'm not sure one way or the other'*, *'I can only make up my mind if similar things happen to me'*, or *'My job is to stay neutral here'*.

Hallucinations

It may also be difficult to elicit discussion of hallucinations because some patients feel embarrassed to mention them and it is uncommon to observe a patient hallucinating in front of you. You should always be on the look out for signs that the patient is hallucinating, eg trying to touch something or speaking to someone who is not there, looking past you, turning the head as if in response to a voice. If this happens ask the patient what is happening. More commonly however, patients do not appear to experience hallucinations during the interview. You should then ask 'probe' questions such as:

- 'Has anything unusual happened to you recently?'
- 'Did you hear voices which no one else can hear?'
- 'Did you ever see things which are strange or that other people cannot see?'

Once established you should ask them to describe the experience, (eg if voices were heard, how many, who was talking, what they were saying, etc, what the experiences mean to the patient, whether or not they are real or arise in the patient's own mind (in the case of voices ask them if they came out of their head or from within) and what has been the effect on the patient.

Common causes of psychoses

Schizophrenia

Unless volunteered by the patient, screen by asking if any strange or unusual things have been happening to them. If psychosis is known about or suspected try to identify positive symptoms, for example:

1 **Bizarre or grandiose delusions**. Common themes of delusions include persecution, bizarre beliefs, grandiosity, other people interfering with thoughts and being controlled by someone.

2 **Hallucinations**. These may be hearing voices which may be giving commands, talking about the person, commenting on actions, repeating thoughts.

3 **First-rank symptoms** of schizophrenia are symptoms which are rare except in schizophrenia and are easily diagnosed by independent observers. They are not the only types of symptoms found in schizophrenia but their presence is highly suggestive of the condition. They are:

- thought possession (insertion, withdrawal, broadcasting)
- passivity phenomena (somatic, thoughts, emotions, acts)
- auditory hallucinations (third person, thought echo, commentary)
- delusional perception.

Mania

Mania is discussed in further detail on page 74 but psychotic ideas in mania are usually mood-congruent in nature, ie grandiose powers, identity or fate. Hallucinations occur less often and can be just as bizarre as those found in schizophrenia. Sometimes it is very difficult to distinguish between schizophrenia and mania on the basis of current symptoms.

Depression

Depression is discussed in further detail on page 71. As in mania, psychotic ideas are mood-congruent, ie delusions of guilt, of the body rotting, of losing money or the home. Persecutory delusions are usually understood by the patient to be the result of something bad that they have (or think they have) done. Auditory hallucinations are more likely to be mood-congruent than in mania.

Dementia

Psychotic features can occur in any form of dementia. Delusions are usually of things being stolen and can be elaborated by believing that someone is breaking into the house. Hallucinations are less well systematised and complex than in other disorders and can be auditory and visual. Lewy body dementia is not uncommon and usually presents with vivid and complex visual hallucinations with relatively well-preserved insight.

Medical conditions

Auditory hallucinations can occur with neurological and systemic conditions such as delirium from any cause, strokes, tumours of the central nervous system, epilepsy or migraine. It can also be caused by various medications, including aspirin toxicity and streptomycin.

Visual hallucinations can be caused by brain tumours (especially of the visual pathway and occipital lobe), delirium, eye disease, migraine, epilepsy or Parkinson's disease treatments especially L-dopa.

Drug-induced psychoses

Common drugs of abuse causing psychoses are amphetamines (causing a schizophrenia-like syndrome), lysergic acid diethylamide (LSD; causing visual hallucinations and secondary paranoia), cannabis (causing paranoid psychoses), ecstasy (paranoid psychosis) and cocaine (delusions of parasitic infestation).

Other causes

Sensory deprivation (eg deafness or poor eyesight) and social isolation increase the chances of hallucinations and delusions.

Practical points

1 **Examiners** and senior colleagues will expect you to know what delusions, hallucinations and first-rank symptoms are. Please refer to pages 40, 48, and 80, respectively, for definitions of each. Learn these off by heart and they will also be very helpful in clinical situations.

2 **Mood changes** with psychotic states can lead to confusion about what the correct diagnosis is. The key is to get a good longitudinal history.

- If mood has clearly changed before the psychosis began then the diagnosis is likely to be depressive psychosis or mania with delusions. In this case the delusions are usually mood-congruent (see page 40) and hallucinations are uncommon and usually auditory.

- If mood changes at the same time as the psychosis emerges then consider the possibility of a schizoaffective disorder.

- If the mood changes after the psychotic ideas emerge then the primary diagnosis is likely to be the primary psychosis (eg schizophrenia or delusional disorder) with a secondary mood disorder (usually depression).

3 Delusions may not be so easy to **diagnose**. In the beginning and towards the end of a psychotic episode delusional ideas may be less firmly held, with the patient being able to consider the possibility that they may be wrong. In this case refer to them as 'emerging' or 'fading' delusions.

4 Always keep in mind the patient's own social, cultural and educational **background**. For example, belief in Voodoo may be appropriate in an individual from Haiti but may not be appropriate to someone born and bred in an English market town. However, if that person from Haiti's beliefs are strange even to people from his own culture then they may still be delusional. If the person from England has had a lifelong interest in the occult then the ideas, though strange, may not be delusional. A good collateral history is important as it will show a decline or a change from the usual in someone who has become psychotic. If you are not familiar with a patient's culture then an opinion from someone from the same culture will be useful.

5 **Hallucinations** are helpful in diagnosing psychotic states.

- Third-person commentary voices are strongly suggestive of schizophrenia.

- Vivid visual hallucinations in clear consciousness are suggestive of organic states, eg Lewy body dementia and drug-induced psychosis.
- Crude hallucinations can occur in delirium, drug-induced states, alcohol withdrawal, etc.

6 **Drug abuse** is an increasingly common cause of psychosis. It is not just younger people who abuse drugs. Unless drug abuse is self-admitted, information from an informant and/or a urinary drug screen will confirm a suspicion. Always try to obtain information via both of these routes.

7 Remember **rarer causes of psychoses**. Delusions without any other symptoms suggest a delusional disorder; in the elderly delusions can be accompanied by auditory or tactile hallucinations and this is sometimes known as paraphrenia (although this diagnosis does not appear in ICD-10).

8 In **dementia** it is unfortunately possible that people (including relatives) actually are stealing from the person. Suspect otherwise if the things reported stolen are trivial, or if the patient claims that the thief enters and leaves without being noticed even if the patient was there.

9 Rarely paranoid delusions may be associated with **an intent to harm people**, eg an imagined persecutor. Rarely hallucinations may 'command' people to attack others. Keep these in mind when assessing risk, though people with mental health problems are far more likely to be attacked than to attack people no matter what tabloid newspapers may have us believe.

10 **Olfactory** hallucinations should always prompt a full neurological assessment.

11 Distinguish delusions from **overvalued ideas**. These are strongly held and may dominate life (and conversation) but are not always illogical or culturally inappropriate. An example is someone preoccupied with the harmful effects of fluoridation of water.

12 Distinguish hallucinations from **pseudo-hallucinations and illusions.**

- *Pseudo-hallucinations* have the vividness of a true perception but the patient knows that they are an internal event, ie insight is retained. Unlike mental imagery patients are unable to dismiss them and they are usually unbidden. Flashbacks in post traumatic stress disorder (PTSD) and the so-called 'widow's hallucination' (see page 50) have these qualities. They can occur in both mental illness and in health especially in situations of stress, tiredness, etc.

- *Illusions* are normal perceptions that are misinterpreted either because of environmental problems (eg poor light) or problems with the patient (eg delirium, poor eyesight, poor hearing, tiredness, extreme emotions, etc).

13 People who are not mentally ill may present with **isolated hallucination** (eg hearing a voice). It is the overall picture which is important and if the person is not distressed, has no other signs of schizophrenia, leads a normal life and has no delusions then there is no mental illness present.

13 The anxious patient

Anxiety is a normal feeling but it becomes a symptom or a disorder when it causes distress, interferes with normal functioning, goes on for too long, or is too intense. Three types of anxiety disorder should be distinguished:

1 **Generalised anxiety** – persistent feelings of anxiety all or most of the time.

2 **Phobic disorders** – anxiety only in response to specific situations, commonly:

- agoraphobia (fear of crowds/open space)
- social phobias (fear of social exposure or scrutiny)
- simple (specific) phobia (fear of single theme, eg spiders).

3 **Panic disorder** – recurrent attacks of severe anxiety which are well-defined and episodic, lasting only a few minutes. These attacks may not be situation-specific.

What to look for

The patient may

1 look worried – tense expression, shaking

2 sound frightened or worried

3 show agitation and over-arousal

4 have signs of autonomic over-activity (dry mouth, tremor, sweating, palpitations, over-breathing, muscle tensions, headache)

5 show behaviour in panic attacks that is severely agitated and apparently bizarre.

What to ask

Generally you should ask what happens, how often, if there is any pattern, any trigger, or anything which makes things better or worse.

1 For **anxiety**:

- feels worried and apprehensive
- irritability
- restlessness
- depersonalisation
- insomnia at the start of the night (initial insomnia)
- psychogenic symptoms such as headache
- memory problems (as a result of information not being registered).

2 For **panic attacks**:

- fear or feeling of threat, panic, or doom that is out of proportion to any perceived danger and cannot be reasoned away, beyond voluntary control
- avoidance of anything that may trigger the panic attacks.
- what triggers it (eg physical exposure, seeing, hearing, imagining it, etc)
- how severe is the panic attack and whether or not there is any anxiety between attacks

3 For **phobias**:

- how often does it happen
- do they avoid these triggers
- do they feel safer at home – are they housebound
- do they need anyone to be with them to feel safe
- what is the effect on their day-to-day life, jobs, relationships, etc.

Practical points

1 The **interview** may be making the patient feel anxious!

2 **Depression** is common – either as a cause, or as a consequence.

3 Remember that **physical causes** for anxiety, especially breathing problems, heart arrhythmias, calcium imbalance and acute intermittent porphyria (rare in real life but strangely common in exams) can give panic attacks.

4 Anxiety can be **secondary** to psychosis (secondary to delusions or hallucinations), dementia (when separated from carer or when cannot cope), and alcohol withdrawal.

5 In **PTSD** anxiety can be generalised as well as specific.

6 Anxiety can occur when **obsessional** symptoms are resisted so screen for these symptoms if appropriate.

7 Anxiety starting for the first time **after the age of 40** usually has an underlying cause.

8 Many patients with anxiety will have a **normal mental state** when interviewed.

14 The obsessive–compulsive patient

Patients with obsessional symptoms may be very pre-occupied with symptoms which, to students, appear bizarre or unbelievable. However, there are important differences compared to the bizarre beliefs experienced by psychotic patients. In particular, patients usually retain insight and understand that their symptoms are senseless. Because psychotic patients accept their delusions as fact, there is no such understanding. Obsessional symptoms can be thoughts, ruminations, ideas, memories and imagery.

Obsessional symptoms are characterised by:

- an intrusive thought, doubt, feeling, or image which is anxiety-provoking or distressing (eg the thought of being dirty, of having left the door unlocked, of wanting to kill a baby, etc)
- the recognition that the thought is your own
- the feeling that such a thought, feeling, etc, is irrational or senseless and unwanted
- trying to resist such thoughts, feelings etc, which usually exacerbates the feeling of distress.

Compulsive acts are recurrent, persistent, often stereotyped actions or rituals that are senseless or unnecessary in themselves or in the number of times they are repeated. Such acts bring temporary relief but may be very disabling, taking a patient several hours to complete.

What to look for

Sometimes people present with the physical signs of an obsessional act, eg raw hands from washing too much.

Obsessional symptoms can occur by themselves or can be part of depression, phobias, hypochondriasis, body image disorders, or organic conditions such as epilepsy, Tourette syndrome and strokes.

What to ask

Ask how often these symptoms happen, whether there is any pattern, whether they arise from within the patient, how long they can be resisted. Ask what the patient does to relieve the distress and what are the consequences of the thoughts or acts (eg wasting time, low mood or difficulty in relationships).

Practical points

1 Obsessional symptoms be **secondary to** part of depression (eg distressing memories) or schizophrenia (eg checking doors repeatedly because of a fear of someone breaking in) and these remit when the primary illness is better. In this case it is better to talk about symptoms rather than a primary disorder.

2 **Differentiate** obsessional symptoms from schizophrenic delusions of thoughts, feelings, etc that are inserted into the patient's mind. The distinguishing feature in obsessional symptoms is that the patient recognises the mental process as their own and often resists the symptoms. Delusions on the other hand are not resisted because they are firmly believed and therefore accepted as fact.

3 People with **PTSD** can have recurrent memories or unbidden imagery and can have rituals to avoid triggering these symptoms. A careful history will reveal the initial trauma and the events, though distressing, are not seen as irrational.

4 People who have **obsessional personality traits** may perform rituals but they do not see these as irrational and it is not performing the ritual that is distressing, rather it is resisting it that causes distress.

15 The patient with post-traumatic stress disorder (PTSD)

Central to all cases of PTSD is a situation where the patient has felt their life was in danger, eg assaults, during wars, natural disasters, accidents, etc. In some professions exposure to these events and their aftermath is more common, eg firemen, police, soldiers, people who have helped during major disasters. Symptoms may emerge a few weeks after the event or years later. The diagnosis may be difficult to pick up because secondary psychiatric illness may be a presenting feature.

What to ask

The general screening questions could be:

'Have you been exposed to frightening events in your life when you felt that you or another person might die or become seriously injured?'

If the answer is yes, then ask *'What was your reaction to this event?'* and *'How did you cope with this event?'*

PTSD cases commonly experience intense fear, horror and helplessness. When assessing patients with PTSD in more detail look for the following.

1 **'Flashbacks'** are usually intrusive and vivid visual images, sometimes described as being like seeing a video of the event in their mind's eye (ie imagery not a hallucination or pseudo-hallucination). Note that flashback symptoms can be in any sensory modality (eg olfactory and somatic flashbacks of burning smells, pain and heat for people who survive a fire).

2 These flashbacks trigger **panic attacks** (and can cause phobic avoidance).

3 **Emotional numbing** causes feelings towards the event and to other people to be impaired and blunted. This may be complained of by family members.

4 **Avoidance** of events/situations which remind the person of the initial trauma.

5 **Nightmares** and sleep disturbance.

6 **Over-arousal** – easily startled, over-vigilant, preoccupation with safety issues (this can shade into paranoia and/or distrust of authority figures).

7 **Depression** – can shade into self-isolation or appear as 'survivor guilt' where the person feels unworthy to have survived and/or feels that they could have done more to save others.

8 **Drug or alcohol abuse** can be caused by underlying symptoms.

Practical points

1 **Symptomatology may be mixed** with other secondary mental health problems.

2 **Avoidance** of painful memories may make the patient less likely to open up or may cause them to minimise the symptoms.

3 **Delayed PTSD** can be triggered by retirement, anniversaries, or new similar events (eg the Gulf War triggering symptoms in Korean War veterans).

4 PTSD symptoms can **range** from single symptoms to full blown illness. Be familiar with the diagnostic criteria.

5 Use open (non-leading) questions when probing for symptoms because PTSD is now a medico-legally significant disorder and there may be pressure on you to diagnose it because of possible **compensation** involved.

6 **Suicide risk** is higher in these patients, partly because the information volunteered by these people is impaired as a result of avoidance and emotional numbing.

16 The confused patient

Confusion is an impairment of the thought process leading to subjective and/or objective signs of befuddlement. It can occur in:

- delirium
- dementia
- schizophrenia
- major depression (can present as 'pseudo-dementia')
- learning difficulties
- intoxication and withdrawal (alcohol, prescribed and non-prescribed drugs)
- mania
- anxiety from any cause.

This section will mainly focus on delirium and dementia.

Delirium (also known as an acute confusional state) is when confusion is acute in onset and reversible and is accompanied by clouding of consciousness.

Dementia (also known as a chronic confusional state) is a progressive irreversible impairment of cognition without any clouding of consciousness. Important sub-types of dementia are mentioned below.

The two conditions can occur together with delirium superimposed on dementia. Indeed, having dementia makes delirium more likely and a less serious medical condition is required to trigger it.

Delirium tremens is the withdrawal stage from alcohol and is characterised by anxiety, agitation, tactile and auditory hallucinations (often crude), visual hallucinations or illusions (often of small images; Lilliputian hallucinations), tachycardia, sweating, tremor, dehydration and raised temperature. This is a medical emergency and needs prompt treatment.

Wernicke's encephalopathy is a triad of ataxia, nystagmus and ophthalmoplegia (usually with clouding of consciousness). It is another alcohol-related emergency which may be prevented by administration of high-dose thiamine to at-risk patients. Wernicke's encephalopathy may lead to Korsakoff syndrome, a disabling and permanent deficit of new long-term memory.

Delirium

Common causes of delirium include infections, prescribed drugs, pain, constipation, metabolic problems (eg hypoglycaemia) and organ failure.

What to look for

1 **Cognitive impairment** – disorientation is a sensitive and early symptom. Disorientation to time is the earliest and most prominent, and less so disorientation to place. There is failure of both registration and recall. The Modified Mini Mental State Examination (3MS; see Appendix 5) is a good way of monitoring fluctuations. If pressed for time or the patient is unco-operative get them to draw a star, interlocking pentagons or a clock face.

2 **Clouding of consciousness** – this fluctuates, becoming especially worse in the evenings and at night, and can range from hypervigilance to stupor. Patients are noticeably very distractible and suggestible.

3 **Abnormalities of perception** – there are hallucinations, misidentifications and illusions (misperceptions). The patient may not to be able to tell the difference between thoughts, memories and normal perceptions.

4 **Abnormalities of affect** – these can range (and often change) from anxiety and irritability to a bemused cheerfulness.

5 **Motor agitation** – this can range from the patient being completely still to profound agitation with unusual energy. Bed-bound patients have been known to get out of bed and walk up whole flights of stairs.

What to ask

It may be very difficult to get the patient to provide a history. In this case concentrate on your observations of the mental state (see above). An informant history is essential to determine the onset of the problems, fluctuations, physical problems at the time of onset, medicines, or drugs taken, etc.

Practical points

1 It is important not just to diagnose delirium but also to determine the **underlying physical cause**. A thorough and systematic physical examination is essential.

2 It is highly unlikely that you will see someone with delirium in an examination but the reverse is true in clinical practice, especially in **hospital settings**.

3 When **interviewing** someone suspected of having dementia, avoid the 'medical model' of questioning. It may be better to start with a discussion of remote events such as childhood experiences, or what the patient did during the war. This approach is less likely to provoke a catastrophic reaction and may help to gain the patient's trust.

Dementia

The three commonest types of dementia are:

1 **Alzheimer's disease**. This is the commonest variety and has a large overlap with the ischaemic end of the vascular dementia spectrum. It is suggested by a gradual and insidious onset in history, relatively well-preserved remote memory and early impairment of language.

2 **Vascular dementia**. There is a spectrum of ischaemic changes ranging from the slow and widespread (the ischaemic end) to the sudden and focal (multi-infarct end). The ischaemic end of the spectrum can present slowly and gradually like Alzheimer's, although there are usually other vascular risk factors. The infarct end of the vascular spectrum presents suddenly with stable periods and decline

after episodes of acute confusion. Neurological signs are common (although usually not as explicit as overt signs of stroke) and memory loss is commonly patchy, including remote memory deficits early on.

3 **Lewy body dementia**. This is the least common of the three and has features of both Alzheimer's and Parkinson's. There are vivid, complex, visual hallucinations, motor features of Parkinson's disease, falls, labile levels of consciousness (changing as quickly as within minutes). This is a diagnosis worth making because patients are very sensitive to the effects of neuroleptics and respond to the anti-dementia drugs.

What to look for

1 **Appearance and behaviour**. The patient may seem self-neglected or may wear clothes incorrectly (eg the wrong way round, inappropriate for the season, etc). You might see purposeless repetitive activity, such as fidgeting, picking at clothes, wandering etc, or the patient might be quiet and motionless. You might also see signs of strokes.

2 **Affect**. Affect may range from unremarkable to suspicious but is commonly bewildered.

3 **Speech**. Speech may be impaired with various degrees of dysphasia – eg words used wrongly (circumlocutions or substitutions) or archaic terms may be used (eg omnibus or wireless). Speech might be repetitive – the same information may be given to you over and over again as if it were being said to you for the first time.

What to ask

During the general part of the questioning (see page 22) record if the patient refers to memory problems at all. If not then start by asking a general question.

'*What has your memory been like recently?*'

Then probe gently any issues that have been raised by either the referee, patient or relative. Do not challenge any assertion that their memory is fine for their age.

Ask the patient and informant specifically about:

- **Pattern of illness** – when started, gradual or sudden start, steady decline or stuttering (stepwise) progression.

- **Cognitive problems** – recent and remote memory loss, difficulty in learning and retaining new material, confabulation, difficulty remembering names or appointments, mislaying things, difficulty expressing themselves (dysphasia), difficulty in dressing, using familiar household items like the television remote control or telephone (dyspraxia).

- **Neuropsychiatric symptoms** – hallucinations, delusions, agitation, aggression, mood changes, apathy, sleep and appetite disturbances.

- **Activities of daily living** – ability to care for self, grooming, dressing, cooking, housework, managing finances, driving, etc.

The rest of the interview is as for elderly people (see page 122). Cognitive assessment is covered in pages 51 and 139 and a standard cognitive assessment is covered in Appendix 5.

Practical points

1 An **informant history** is essential. Ask the informant beforehand if they want to speak to you before or after the patient interview as some people feel uncomfortable discussing their relative's memory problems in front of them. An informant needs to be present when the patient is interviewed.

2 **Apparent cognitive difficulties** can also occur when the patient is angry, unco-operative, or suffering from any difficulties with hearing or vision, any difficulties with speech and poor level of general education.

3 Patients who have a **high level of education** may perform well despite having cognitive impairment.

4 Sometimes it is difficult to distinguish dementia from depressive **pseudo-dementia**; re-testing cognition after a good course of anti-depressants or ECT may be the only way to tell them apart.

5 You may not be able to get explicit **consent** for the interview from a patient with dementia. Record this in your interview and it will help if the relative or informant's wishes are then recorded instead (although they cannot consent on the patient's behalf).

6 When probing for memory loss the patient might be unconcerned or might become very irritable and refuse to answer any further questions. If an informant is present the demented patient often keeps looking to their relative to answer questions for them, eg how old they are, when did their spouse die, etc. Make a note of this and try to get the patient to attempt the answer first and then ask the relative to give you the correct answer. The reason for this is that a **depressed patient** will more often say 'I don't know' if pressed. You would not pick this up if the relative is answering the questions.

7 An **apparent sudden start to memory loss** might be the sudden 'decompensation' of someone who had already had memory loss for some time when placed in a new situation like going on holiday, having a spouse die, or moving house.

17 The mute patient

Distinguish simple mutism (not saying anything) and stupor (where mutism is combined with no movement or action at all (akinesia). Possible causes of mutism include:

- stupor (akinetic mutism) as a result of severe depression, mania, or schizophrenia
- specific neurological causes (eg epilepsy, stroke, neuroleptic malignant syndrome)
- effect of drugs or alcohol
- distraction as a result of delusions/hallucinations or thought crowding
- dissociative states (conversion disorder)
- catatonic schizophrenia
- malingering
- learning disability.

What to look for

A comprehensive physical examination, including plantar responses, reflexes and cranial nerves, should be performed. If neurological examination is unremarkable and the patient is immobile, then consider stupor. People in stupor are usually very aware of their surroundings and will be able to hear you but not to respond. There may be few clues as to the cause other than an informant's history. Stupor can lead to dehydration and pressure sores if not promptly treated.

Mobile individuals may exhibit motor signs of catatonia including:

- increased muscle tone
- waxy flexibility
- psychological pillow or other bizarre postures
- excitement
- echopraxia.

What to ask

If there is no evidence of catatonic motor signs, persevere with a few simple questions, leaving a long interval between questions. This may reveal extreme psycho-motor retardation, as sometimes seen in depression. If the patient remains mute, re-assess after a short interval. Exceptionally, mute patients may need to be admitted for observation. Try to identify an informant and obtain a history of recent events and check for any past psychiatric history.

Practical points

1 An **informant history** is essential when assessing a mute patient.

2 It is very important to consider and exclude **organic causes** of mutism. For example, non-convulsive status epilepticus or herpes simplex encephalitis are causes of mutism that must be treated promptly. Lowering of consciousness strongly suggests an organic cause but severe psychomotor retardation may mimic that. If in doubt ask for a neurological or medical opinion. Investigations such as computed tomography, magnetic resonance imaging, electroencephalogram etc should also be considered.

18 The angry patient

Anger and violence can occur in normal people and are not necessarily a sign of mental illness. However, anger can occur in the following psychiatric situations:

- mania or hypomania
- any disorder with persecutory ideation (eg drug intoxication, chronic alcoholism, schizophrenia, dementia)
- delirium (especially drug- or alcohol-withdrawal, hypoglycaemia, encephalitis, after a head injury, or after an epileptic fit)
- anti-social or borderline personality disorder.

What to look for

Many violent episodes are predictable. The clues that a patient is becoming aggressive include:

- glaring at you
- muscle tension, resulting in tremor
- increased agitation and arousal
- a change in posture, such as leaning towards you, clenching fists, jabbing finger in air at you
- signs of autonomic over-activity, eg facial flushing or blanching, shaking
- not paying any attention to questions
- invasion of your personal space
- verbal aggression or aggression to objects
- misinterpretation of what is being said as aggressive or derogatory.

What to ask

If you do not feel uneasy or at risk, try to defuse the situation by initially commenting on the fact that they are angry, acknowledge that everyone has the right to feel angry and explain that you are there to try to help them. Allow time for ventilation of their feelings and lots of personal space (without appearing to be frightened or angry yourself).

If this fails or if behaviour becomes inappropriate without being directly threatening try to point out what behaviour or language is unacceptable, eg that it is not a good idea to let their feelings run away with them etc. At this point you should start making plans to leave and/or summon help. To leave safely, give a reason for stopping the interview, and back out of the room.

Do not turn your back on someone who could be, or is already becoming, aggressive.

Practical points

1 Do not try to use **logic** with people who are intoxicated (either alcohol or drugs) or delirious. Repeat reassurances using simple and neutral words. Keep out of their personal space.

2 **Do not get angry** yourself – the patient may be trying to provoke you to justify a physical attack.

3 Do not forget to check the patient's **blood glucose and alcohol** levels if you can.

19 The patient with alcohol-related problems

Alcohol abuse is a common problem. It may be a cause of, a contributing factor to, or a consequence of mental illness. It is an important risk factor in suicidal behaviour and has serious physical consequences. There are three levels of pathology, shown below, and the progression between each is not clear cut.

Excessive drinking ➔
Drinking alcohol is in excess of safe limits
(21 units/week in men and 14 units/week in women)

Problem drinking ➔
Excessive drinking with adverse consequences
(see below)

Alcohol dependency
Excessive drinking with physical and psychological dependency

There are seven features in the history which characterise full-blown dependence.

1 **Stereotyped pattern** of drinking. Drinking is not in response to usual cues (eg celebration) but to avoid withdrawal symptoms.

2 **Primacy** of drink-seeking behaviour. Drinking goes on despite adverse consequences.

3 Increased **tolerance** to alcohol. Increasing quantities of drink are needed to produce intoxication.

4 Repeated **withdrawal** symptoms. When blood alcohol levels become low – usually in the morning, but mild symptoms, such as anxiety, tremor and sweating, may be present throughout the day.

5 Repeated **relief drinking**. Keeps these mild symptoms from turning into full-blown delirium tremens.

6 Subjective awareness of **compulsion** to drink. The desire to drink is seen as irrational, and is resisted but ultimately given in to (and sometimes followed by intense guilt feelings).

7 **Relapse after abstinence**. Patients return to drinking at the level they had been at before stopping very rapidly after restarting.

What to look for

Unless the patient is drunk when you see him then look for signs of chronic alcohol abuse. The apparently normal person may conceal a serious alcohol problem and the stereotype, eg dishevelled tramp with a bulbous red nose and a bottle of cheap cider in a brown paper bag, is rare.

What to ask

An alcohol history must include the following:

1 **What is drunk** (beer, spirits, cider, etc)? Always probe for other types of drink than the one first volunteered by the patient. Try to quantify in units (one unit is equivalent to one-half pint of weak beer or lager, one pub measure of spirits (usually much smaller than those poured at home) or one small glass of wine; some strong lagers may be double the strength of ordinary lager).

2 **How much** is drunk and how much money is spent per week?

3 **How often**? (usual consumption a week is a useful measure)

4 **Where**? (in pub, at home, at work, etc)

5 **When** does drinking start during the day?

6 What are **triggering** factors? (availability of alcohol, current stresses)

7 Are there **binges** and/or steady drinking?

8 When did drinking **start**?

9 What was longest period when **abstinent**?

10 Was **help** sought in the past? (Alcoholics Anonymous, counsellors, detoxification units, etc)

11 What are **predisposing factors**? (family history of alcoholism)

12 **Complications**:

- *Psychological.* Irritability and violence, anxiety, depression, palimpsest (transient reversible memory lapses for recent events), blackouts, alcoholic hallucinosis (voices in setting of clear consciousness), deliberate self-harm, morbid jealousy.

- *Physical.* Acute intoxication, anorexia, nausea, diarrhoea, retching, gastritis, ulcers, hepatitis, cirrhosis and jaundice, memory loss, peripheral neuropathy. Delirium tremens is precipitated by withdrawal. Someone with delirium tremens is confused, may have crude auditory hallucinations (eg noises) or complex visual ones (eg the classic pink elephants), ataxia, paranoia, fits, and the mood is usually one of intense fear.

- *Interpersonal.* Break-up of relationships, alienation of helping networks.

- *Work.* Loss of job, days off sick, poor performance at work, accidents at work.

- *Social.* Drink driving or public disorder offences.

- *Economic.* Debts, selling possessions, no relation between money spent on alcohol and income.

If the patient is suspected of having a drink problem and alcohol abuse is suspected then two screening questionnaires are useful.

The **CAGE** questionnaire is a useful screening questionnaire to ask when alcohol abuse is suspected:

- Have you ever felt you wanted to **C**ut down on your drinking?

- Has anyone ever **A**nnoyed you by criticising your drinking?

- Have you ever felt **G**uilty about your drinking?

- Have you had an '**E**ye opener'? (a drink first thing in the morning to avoid withdrawal symptoms).

Mayfield, D et al 'The CAGE questionnaire: validation of a new alcoholism instrument' *American Journal of Psychiatry*, 131:1121–1123 (1974)

If two or more answers are positive you must take a full alcohol history. CAGE is easy to remember but tends to pick up only the more severe end of drinking problems.

An alternative (and more sensitive) screening questionnaire is **AUDIT** provided in Appendix 6 in its short form. AUDIT probes alcohol consumption, features of dependence and harm resulting from drinking. There are 10 questions. Each question is scored from 0 to 4. A score of 8 in men and 7 in women indicates a strong likelihood of hazardous or harmful alcohol consumption.

Practical points

1   An **informant history** is important, especially in cases where the history is unclear, the patient is thought to be underestimating their intake and where family or friends are being affected by the drinking.

2   An alcohol history should always be supplemented by a **physical investigation** (see page 60) and blood tests for red blood cell volume, Gamma glutamytransferase (γGT) and carbohydrate transferin test which are suggestive of acute and chronic alcohol abuse, respectively.

20 The substance misuser

It is not possible to cover drug abuse in detail in this book but some basic information will be given to point the assessor in the right direction. Remember people often use more than one drug.

Drug (route)	Effects	Withdrawal	Other effects
Morphine **Heroin** **Methadone** (can be injected, sniffed, or smoked)	Euphoria Reduction in pain Drowsiness Loss of appetite	Agitation Irritability Insomnia Hot and cold flushes Dizziness Pain, especially in back and legs Enlarged pupils Piloerection	Abuser may have lost weight (so called heroin chic) Small pupils Lack of co-ordination Dry mouth Constipation May have injection marks and thrombosed veins May have signs of hepatitis and human immunodeficiency virus infection
LSD (ingested)	Depends on setting and mood but includes: Synaesthesia (senses become mixed up) Illusions and hallucinations Mystical or ecstatic feelings Panic attacks Depression Disorientation (three in 'bad trips')	No effects	Flashbacks may occur up to many months later Schizophrenia may be precipitated in vulnerable individuals Accidents whilst in use may be mistaken for suicide attempts
Amphetamine (ingested or injected)	Increased arousal vigilance, increased energy, wakefulness confidence and well-being Prolonged use can lead to weight loss and a schizophrenia-like psychosis	Prolonged sleep and extreme lethargy Irritability Depression Distress	Dilated pupils Irregular and fast heart beat Can become aggressive especially in overdose Can be mistaken for hypomania or schizophrenia

Drug	Effects	Withdrawal/after effects	Signs and complications
Cocaine (sniffed, chewed, smoked or injected)	Depends on route but includes as for amphetamines but also: Euphoria; Increased sexual desires; Weight loss; Perceptual disturbances including tactile hallucinations	Depression; Exhaustion; Paranoia	Perforated nasal septa and chronic rhinitis can be signs of chronic abuse; Can have tachycardia and dilated pupils
Ecstasy (ingested)	Depends on dose and mood; Feeling of well-being; Increased confidence; Increased heart rate and blood pressure; Anxiety; Nausea; Loss of appetite; Paranoid feelings; Hallucinations in high doses	Hangover; Sleep problems; Irritability	Tooth clenching and dry mouth may be observed; Rhabdomyolysis, renal failure and sudden death have been reported
Marijuana (smoked or ingested)	Slowing down; Impaired memory and thinking (daydreaming); Giggling; Anxiety and even frank paranoia; Tachycardia; Depression and lack of motivation; Increased hunger for sweet foods	Irritability; Sleeplessness; Restlessness	User has bloodshot eyes; Can increase chances of developing or precipitating schizophrenia
Solvents (sniffed as an aerosol or inhaled in bags)	Depending on solvent-use can cause: Confusion; Hallucinations and delusions; Euphoria; Slurred speech	Anxiety; Agitation; Crude auditory hallucinations; Tremor	Can have neurological or cardiac damage; May accidentally suffocate with head in bag (and can be mistaken for a suicide attempt)

21 The patient with an eating disorder

Eating disorders are uncommon but can be difficult to spot. The patient may present with secondary physical problems, with declining performance at school, or a poor relationship with the family.

Anorexia nervosa is a failure to eat enough, resulting in weight loss. It is most common in young women though it is found in men and even older people (either as a new case or in someone who has had anorexia since they were young). It is more common in Western cultures. People at high risk include those from higher social classes, high achievers (eg in students, athletes, fashion models, or ballerinas), people with obsessional traits and those whose family seems over controlling. It commonly starts in adolescence.

Bulimia is binge eating followed by purging using laxatives or self-induced vomiting, and can exist by itself or be part of anorexia nervosa.

Anorexia

What to ask

The SCOFF questionnaire* screens for eating disorders. It asks the following questions:

1 *'Do you make yourself **S**ick because you feel uncomfortably full?'*

2 *'Do you worry that you have lost **C**ontrol over how much you eat?'*

3 *'Have you recently lost more than **O**ne stone in a 3-month period?'*

* Morgan, J.F., Reid, F., Lacey, J.H. 1999 The SCOFF questionnaire: assessment of a new screening tool for eating disorder. *British Medical Journal*, 319, 1467–1468.

4 *'Do you believe yourself to be **F**at when others say you are too thin?'*

5 *'Would you say **F**ood dominates your life?'*

Two or more positive answers indicate a likely case of anorexia or bulimia. In addition probe for:

- **Weight phobia** – overvalued ideas about shape and weight. There is intense loathing of obesity and weight gain. These attitudes are extreme, inflexible, and any suggestion of a weight gain is seen as a frightening threat. This reaches delusional intensity but given Western cultural values is not very much out of keeping with cultural norms and ideas about perfect body weight.

- **Body image disturbance** – ask what is seen as an ideal body weight. Actual misperception of one's body size is rare and disparagement (or hatred) of one's body is more common. People who are emaciated still believe they are too fat.

- **Hormonal disturbance** – amenorrhoea (primary or secondary) is essential in diagnosis of anorexia in women; a menstrual history should be taken.

- **Denial** is very common and patients often try to hide signs and symptoms.

- **Mood** is very labile and depression is very common.

- **Obsessional symptoms** may be present, often to do with food. A key feature of anorexia is the fear of losing control over weight. Sometimes there is an unusual degree of interest in food, recipes, calorie content, etc. Calorie counting of food is common. The obsessional behaviour can extend to other areas, eg cleanliness, housework, etc.

What to look for

Some people with anorexia may wear loose clothing to disguise their weight loss. Try to perform a physical examination whenever possible and look out for:

- enlarged salivary glands

- pubic and axillary hair may not have developed (if illness started before puberty)
- breast atrophy if illness started after puberty
- skin looks rough, dry and aged (although the overall appearance may be of someone younger)
- low blood pressure and slow pulse
- extremities cold, blue and oedematous
- nutritional myopathy (muscle wasting but good power and intact reflexes)
- weight must be least 15% below expected weight for age and sex (body mass index is 17.5 or less).

Bulimia

The general psychopathology resembles that of anorexia (persistent concern with food, body shape and weight, depression, obsessionality, etc).

What to ask

You also need an informant to verify the history given by the patient. Look for:

- **Recurrent binge eating**. Of any food but commonly 'forbidden food' which does not have to be cooked. The amount of food eaten during a binge may be very large. Exhaustion, vomiting, abdominal distension, interruption, or running out of food will stop a binge. There is a feeling of lack of control over eating behaviour during binges.
- **Weight-loss behaviour**. Involves self-induced vomiting and laxative, diuretic or even amphetamine abuse.
- **Depression**. Strict dieting, fasting or vigorous exercise often follows bingeing, with feelings of depression, guilt and self-disgust. Patients sometimes shop-lift (commonly food) or abuse alcohol because of their low mood.

What to look for

As for anorexia but also:

- body weight can be normal, or even overweight, unless it presents as part of anorexia (see above)

- calluses may be present on back of hand from repeated self-induced vomiting (Russell's sign)

- inside enamel of teeth may be worn from repeated vomiting

- occasionally there is enlargement of the parotid salivary glands.

Practical points

1 You need an **informant**, ideally one who knows and lives with the patient, because much of the time the anorectic patient will deny problems and hide the signs from everyone.

2 Not only is **denial** common but patients actively hide their low weight (eg putting stones in their pockets when getting weighed).

3 If the patient has **children** their preoccupation with food may extend to them so it is important to review the weight of the children as well.

4 Secondary **depression** is common and some people seem to try to commit suicide by taking their dieting to extremes.

5 A **family assessment** is helpful so refer to a family assessment unit.

6 Rarely **oesophageal tears** may result from the repeated vomiting so look out for any sudden retrosternal pain and/or blood being spat out.

SECTION D

Interviewing Specific Groups of Patients

22 Assessing children and adolescents

Julia Gledhill

Preparing for the interview

Anticipating which family members will arrive for a first appointment is difficult. Provide enough chairs for everyone. Seeing where people sit gives useful information, eg in a family where parents argue a lot, the child may seat themselves between the mother and father; a father excluded from the mother–child relationship may sit at a distance.

Make the room inviting by having age-appropriate toys and drawing materials on display (and letting the child know they can use them). A small table and chair are useful. Particularly helpful are toys which easily tell a story, eg dolls house, model animals, toy cars. Children are used to playing; this helps them feel comfortable and provides 'props' to help you understand how they are feeling, eg asking a child to tell you about their drawing.

Children generally live with families and attend school. Information from parents and school (with consent) usually forms an integral part of the assessment.

Meeting a child psychiatrist may be novel for children and families. It is helpful to hear their understanding of why they have come to see you. Introducing yourself and explaining your job are also essential. A possible statement would be: *'I am a doctor. My special job is to help children with their worries and troubles. I spend time listening to and speaking with children and Mummies and Daddies to try to help children worry less and make life easier for them at home and at school.'*

Establishing a good rapport from the start is of paramount importance. Five minutes talking generally, eg about a favourite football team, helps the child to relax and start talking. It also demonstrates your interest in them. If the child is aware of difficulties, it is helpful to find out how (s)he views the problem(s).

Match the complexity of language used to the stage of cognitive development of the individual child or adolescent. Use shorter sentences with younger children. In addition, find out words that may be specific to that child or family, for example:

> interviewer [to the mother of a young child (David)]:
> '. . . and what does David call his grandmother?'
> mother: 'He has always called her "Nana".'

Obtaining the history and examining the child's mental state

Who to talk to

Often the whole family is seen together initially but it is often useful to also see the child alone.

Explain the structure of the meeting at the outset, eg for a school age child say, 'I'm going to talk to the whole family first and then I'd like to spend a little bit of time with you by yourself if that's OK;... if you like, we can play and draw while we talk; Mummy and Daddy will wait downstairs in the waiting room where you sat when you first got here and then we'll ask them to come back in and we'll all talk together before we finish today.'

Some history will be obtained from parent(s) and some from the child (information from parents is generally greater for younger children).

The observations by both parents and teachers of the child's mental state should be considered, in addition to direct examination of the child.

Parents may be more aware of a child's externalising symptoms, eg tantrums, hyperactivity, stealing, but are less accurate in their reports of emotional symptoms, eg hopelessness, worries, guilt, suicidal thoughts.

It often helps to see the child alone. This is less anxiety-provoking if the child has first been interviewed with its parents. If the child sees that the whole family are happy to talk to you then they should feel more confident when alone. Do let the child know where his/her parents are waiting to reduce anxiety.

See parents independently as well. If the child is too young to wait alone ask families in advance to bring someone with them for this purpose. Alternatively, parents may be invited for a subsequent appointment without the child.

History and Mental State Examination

In general, this is less systematic than for adults.

Especially in younger children topics are rarely covered in a pre-determined order. Akin to physical examination of a child, information may be indirectly offered at different times in the interview or may usefully be opportunistically elicited, eg if a parent is talking about their own depressed mood, this may be an appropriate time to ask, *'Mummy's been telling me about times when she feels sad. Can you tell me about times when you feel sad?'*

Mental state examination of children is probably more reliant on observation during the course of the meeting than on the specific enquiry that is more usual for adults. For example an adolescent who is distressed and clingy at a request to separate from his/her mother for an individual assessment may suggest separation anxiety. Cognitive abilities can be assessed from the child's speech and play.

Generally use open rather than closed questions, eg *'All children feel sad at some time or other. What sort of things make you sad?'* rather than *'Do you feel sad sometimes?'*

However, if the child is very unforthcoming, it can sometimes be helpful to offer the child alternatives, eg *'Are you worried about wetting yourself at home* **or** *at school* **or** *somewhere else?'* This helps the child feel that you understand what his/her concerns may be and facilitates later elaboration. Supplementary questions may be needed to clarify the answer.

A useful question to gain a deeper understanding of a child's perspective is *'If you could have three wishes, what would they be?'* This helps reveal the child's concerns which they may have been unable to articulate on direct questioning and can later elaborate on.

Never forget that even if children appear completely engrossed in play, they will be listening to the conversation and may respond to it, eg if a depressed parent starts crying, the child may change his/her play to something (s)he feels is entertaining, trying to make the parent laugh or the child may stop playing and try to comfort their parent. This gives clues to patterns of interaction at home.

Considerations for different age groups

Children

- Adjust **vocabulary** and **interviewing style** to reflect the cognitive ability of the child. The concentration span of children may be limited eg young children up to 7 may become distractible quickly and the first individual assessment should be restricted to no more than 15–20 mins. Older children may cope with a longer available.

- Be clear about what you are asking and **give cues**, eg a young child will not understand 'a day', 'a week' etc as adults do. 'A long time' may have a different meaning for children and adults. Therefore use tangible cues, eg 'at supper time', 'when you are at nursery'.

- Do not sit opposite the child repeatedly asking questions as you would with an adult. **Encourage the child to play** with the toys and draw; talk to them about what they are doing and while engaged in these activities, gently try to gain the information you want, eg *'... the little boy in your picture looks a bit sad. What sort of things make you sad?'*

- *Play materials should be age-appropriate.*

Adolescents

The interviewing style for adolescents is more similar to that used in adults; adolescents (in contrast to younger children) think less concretely and are more able to use abstract thinking. Adolescents are usually seen on their own. If a parent seems reluctant to leave the room, it is helpful to say 'I usually see teenagers on their own so I wonder if you would mind waiting outside for about 20 minutes.'

- Issues of **confidentiality** need to be considered and the 'ground rules' explained to the adolescent, eg *'I'm going to talk with you to find out what's been happening from your point of view and to see how you are feeling about things. I will not repeat what we say word for word to your parents, but when we have finished talking, we will ask your parents to join us and it may be helpful, if you agree, for us to think with them about some of the things that crop up. However, if something comes up during our conversation that I am very worried about because I think you are in danger or at risk in some way, it would be wrong of me to ignore that and we will talk together about what we might do and who we need to talk to. We may need to share something like that with your parents.'*

- This may be an adolescent's **first experience** of being interviewed in this way. Time spent building a rapport (chatting about things which interest them) at the start may yield later gains in terms of the amount and quality of information elicited. Adolescents are often relieved to know a psychiatrist is interested in listening to them.

- Adolescents (and younger children) may feel they are the only person with a particular problem so it is often helpful to '**normalise**' their experience to encourage them to be more forthcoming, eg *'Most teenagers feel depressed from time to time. Have there been times in the last few weeks when you have felt down?'*

Evaluating symptomatology

To assess the pathological significance of symptoms the following points should be considered.

1. the degree of suffering the symptoms are causing the child and their parents

2. any resulting functional impairment, particularly with regard to three domains:

   - school performance and behaviour
   - peer relationships and leisure activities
   - family relationships.

For example anxiety just prior to a school exam is usually not a cause for concern but several hours of worry (from which the child cannot be distracted) each day about exams which impairs their concentration (and academic attainment) and sleep is more likely to be of significance.

Diagnoses

The same diagnostic criteria (ICD-10 and the fourth revision of the Diagnostic and Statistical Manual of Mental Disorders (DSM-IV)) are used for disorders occurring in all age groups. However, some disorders are more common in specific age groups, eg psychotic disorders are uncommon in childhood but more frequent in adolescence, and the symptoms of specific disorders may differ between children and adults, eg for major depressive episode (DSM-IV), the prominent mood change may be irritability, not depression.

In addition, ICD-10 and DSM-IV include specific diagnoses which usually have their onset in childhood or adolescence, eg enuresis, separation anxiety.

Summary

- Children are usually assessed with their family and/or alone. Parents are often seen independently. Some child psychiatrists always like to see the whole family together.

- The assessment takes longer than in adults.

- More time needs to be spent with introductions, familiarisation and building rapport.

- Less time is spent on direct questioning.

- There is greater emphasis on indirect information gathering from observations and assimilation of what children say and do during the meeting.

23 Assessing the elderly

The psychiatric assessment of older people involves all the skills used in the assessment of younger people. There are changes of emphasis, however:

- The presentation of the illness may be different, eg agitation is a common problem in older depressed people, and older people presenting with schizophrenia tend to have fewer negative symptoms.
- The epidemiology of disorders differs. Dementia is rare below the age of 65 years.
- Older people have more physical morbidity and social needs. They are often lonely and isolated.

Preparing for the interview

The following factors need to be considered when interviewing the elderly patient.

- **Location** – the interview is best done at home; older people find it hard to travel, and seeing someone at home can provide invaluable information on levels of self-care.
- **Informant** – the input of an informant is more important in the elderly, especially in cases of dementia, and ideally the informant should be the main care-giver (if relevant). It is therefore best to arrange beforehand for an informant to be present.
- **Referral information** – more emphasis needs to be placed on physical health and drugs taken.
- **Informant** – If there is time and there is no information on the referral letter, check if the patient has insight into their problem. If they do not then they might be upset at the information an informant might want to give you. Ask the informant if they feel the information they have can be discussed with the informant freely in front of the patient. If both feel that a discussion should take place without the

patient being present, make a separate appointment before seeing your patient.

The interview

Obtaining the history

- Many older people appreciate a respectful **interest** in their life.
- Speak to both the patient and the **informant**. It may sometimes be better to speak to people separately.
- **Hearing** difficulties may be present, and hearing aids may get switched off.
- Use a **slower pace** for the interview; the person may be slower (with memory problems or expressive difficulties) and may have more to say (in terms of a longer life history).
- Do not forget **alcohol** problems – drug abuse is not yet a common difficulty but will become so as younger generations age.
- Retain a **holistic** view. Physical health is crucial to mental health, think how services can help. A systemic enquiry about falls, breathing, chest pain, dizziness, etc is important.
- Consider **iatrogrenic** problems. What drugs are being taken is important (there can be problems with polypharmacy and drug side-effects).
- Assess **finances**. Poverty is common in the elderly so check if finances are adequate. Consider enduring power of attorney or referral to the Court of Protection as appropriate.
- Remember **risk**. There may be abuse by a family member, strangers, or in an institution.
- Identify **supportive networks**. These may be:
    - family, friends, neighbours
    - Churches, voluntary groups, social clubs, day centres
    - home helps, meals on wheels, district nurses.

Mental state

In the elderly patient it is important to take the following into consideration.

- Remember expressive and receptive dysphasias may be present that will hamper history-taking.

- Watch for consistency and accuracy of the patient's account. Patients with dementia may initially seem plausible, and problems may only emerge after several minutes of interviewing. Patients with dementia may start to repeat themes as if they were telling them for the first time.

- If dementia is suspected, screen for hallucinations and delusions, dangerous behaviour (eg leaving the gas on, flooding the house, wandering at night, getting lost, etc).

- All older patients require a comprehensive cognitive assessment.

Physical health

Assess general physical health, such as pulse rate, nutrition, dentition, dehydration, ulcers, etc, see page 60 for more details.

Carer needs

Remember that carers may have mental health and physical health problems of their own. Assess the role of any carers:

1 What is done, how often

2 What effect does caring have on their relationship (eg do they resent it?)

3 Effects on health (mental and physical), social life, income.

Environment

Assess the **home environment**. Observe stairs, heating, security, food in the cupboard and fridge, cleanliness, clutter, etc.

Observe the **neighbourhood**

- shops, buses
- access to the neighbourhood (stairs etc).

Summary

- People in the late part of their lives are facing end-of-life issues and existential concerns – they may be reflecting on what sort of a life have they had.
- In all older people, the psychological, social, physical and environmental needs require assessment.

24 Assessing people with learning difficulties

Sally-Ann Cooper

Adults with learning difficulties have a higher prevalence of psychiatric disorders compared with the general population, and can experience all types. All of the components of psychiatric assessment used for the general population should be included when assessing an adult with learning difficulties, together with the additional considerations outlined below.

Communication

The psychiatrist is responsible for enabling an effective communication process.

- The **setting** and **developmental abilities** of the person with learning disabilities should be considered.

- **Familiar environments** are preferable where possible, free from noise and interruption, and the person may benefit from support from someone they know well. It is important to use developmentally appropriate language, and to be aware of acquiescence and suggestibility.

- Non verbal cues such as intonation, gesture, bodily posture and movement, pictures and symbols can all contribute to communication, as well as spoken words.

Informants

It is always essential to take the person's history from one or more informants as well as listening to their own account. Even a person with mild learning disabilities is likely to experience difficulties in providing their own full psychiatric history, eg with temporal sequencing of events.

- Family carers usually know and understand their relative with learning disabilities extremely well, and can provide detailed and accurate information, including noticing quite subtle changes in behaviour.

- Sometimes this is also the case for paid carers, depending upon the length of time the paid carer has known the person, the amount of individual and shared time they spend with the person, and how well information is communicated between different members of the carer-team, among other factors.

- When the person with learning disabilities lives with paid support, it is always important to also contact any living relatives to secure details regarding background history, and also to obtain current information from the relative if they are still in contact.

A developmental approach

As well as assessing biological, psychological and social dimensions, the developmental dimension should be included in the examination.

1 Determine the cause of the person's learning disabilities, their current adaptive skill level, and development through their life.

2 The cause of learning disabilities may help to understand the person's current presentation, eg through knowledge of the associated behavioural phenotype (such as Down syndrome with dementia and depression), and also any differential diagnoses requiring exclusion, eg physical problems commonly associated with specific genetic syndromes.

3 Assessment of adaptive skill level is important, as psychopathology is interpreted within the context of the person's ability level.

Psychopathology

1 **Pathoplasticity**. Psychopathology within psychiatric disorders differs at different developmental levels. For

example, a developmental age of about seven years is required to understand the concept of guilt, which will never be achieved by a person with severe or profound learning disabilities. Hence, guilt will not be a feature of depressive illness at this level. Conversely, irritable mood, reduced communication, social withdrawal and loss of skills are common features of a depressive episode, together with sleep and appetite disturbance.

2 **State versus trait**. Assessment of each item of psychopathology should be set within the context of what is usual for that person, to differentiate symptoms from long-standing traits.

- Some people with learning disabilities have long-standing traits which are usual for them and so not indicative of psychiatric illness, eg sleep disturbance.

- Sometimes long standing problem behaviours can be reduced when the person is unwell with psychiatric illness, eg morbid-overeating may reduce in a person with Prader–Willi syndrome during a depressive episode.

- More typically, however, problem behaviours are increased during discrete episodes of psychiatric illness.
  Long-standing problem behaviours not related to psychiatric illness also require proper assessment to determine their aetiology. This includes assessing frequency, severity, duration and chronicity, and associated factors (including antecedents and consequences of behaviour, in addition to relationships to biological factors, and relevant findings from the personal, social and developmental history).

3 **Developmental disorders with superimposed psychiatric illness**. Some people have additional developmental disorders, such as autistic spectrum disorders or attention deficit and hyperactivity disorder. They can acquire

additional psychiatric illness and hence assessment of each item of psychopathology must be within the context of what is developmentally the norm for that person.

4 **Selectivity in volunteered carer information**. Carers are more likely to tell you about problems which pose an immediate management problem or a risk, such as aggression, destructiveness and self-injury, and are less likely to spontaneously report eg social withdrawal and reduced communication. Therefore, always conduct a comprehensive review of all possible psychopathology.

Epilepsy

About 25% of people with learning disabilities experience epilepsy, which is therefore an important differential in the psychiatric diagnosis, eg between panic attacks and complex partial seizures. Some of the side-effects of anti-epileptic drugs can mimic psychiatric disorder, eg depressive episode, and therefore should also be considered in differential diagnosis. Psychotropic drugs can affect seizure threshold and anti-epileptic drugs can affect mental state.

Other physical health needs

Other physical health needs occur more commonly in people with learning disabilities than the general population.

- Some are specifically associated with certain genetic syndromes, eg Down syndrome with thyroid disorder and sensory impairments.

- Some are more common at more severe levels of learning disabilities, eg gastro-oesophageal reflux disorder.

- People who have limited verbal communication skills often cannot describe symptoms, and so presentations include changes in behaviour and the onset of problem behaviours such as aggression and sleep disturbance. As these may be confused as symptoms of psychiatric illness, it is important to consider physical health needs and pain within the differential diagnosis, as well as drug side-effects.

Personal history

Many of today's adults and older adults with learning disabilities did not have the usual childhood opportunities and securities afforded the majority of the population:

- many adults with learning disabilities were raised in institutions
- they have experienced a repeated pattern of broken relationships through staff changes
- abuse, neglect, bullying, harassment and exploitation have been common
- having a family member with learning disabilities may change the family dynamics.

These factors may all be relevant to a person's current psychiatric state.

Social history

Not everyone living in the community experiences social integration and inclusion.

- The cost of living can be higher for people with disabilities (eg transport costs) and employment opportunities may be limited.
- Poverty of environment, social relationships and networks may impact upon health.
- Life events for people with learning disabilities often occur in multiples, eg the death of a parent may also result in a move to temporary accommodation, dislocation from a familiar neighbourhood and neighbours, change in day centre and the appearance of new carers.

It is therefore important that all of these factors are included in the psychiatric assessment.

Mental state examination

It is possible to get a person with learning disabilities who has delusions to agree with you that they are not true – temporarily, until you stop actively persuading her/him. A depressed person with learning disabilities can be encouraged to smile and laugh at your joke if you model this for her/him. These issues are similar to the acquiescence and suggestibility that can be found in verbal communication. It is important to be aware of this if significant signs are not to be overlooked in the mental state examination.

Summary

It takes longer to complete a comprehensive psychiatric assessment with an adult with learning disabilities than with a person of average ability, as there are more elements to it. Informants are essential. If undertaken competently, the gains for the person with learning disabilities can be considerable.

25 Assessing people with an ethnic minority background

Dinesh Bhugra

Black and ethnic minority individuals form around 6% of the population in the UK although the population in metropolitan cities may reach up to 26% in some parts, eg in some boroughs of London. The epidemiological data shows that the rates of some mental illnesses are higher in some groups. Culture is defined as beliefs, behaviours and meanings which may be transmitted across generations and are imbibed by the individual from a number of sources. Cultures may produce, protect from, or modify mental ill health. Thus the role of culture in defining and understanding abnormality is crucial.

Principles of assessment

Some of the factors discussed below are common to all groups and others are specific to black and ethnic minority patients.

Understanding cultural factors

Understanding the culture is important in three ways:

- **Assessing the world view**. Often the way in which individuals make sense of their world and how it is imbued with meaning will influence the way they perceive the distress, the way this distress is expressed and how these are affected by culture. Culture influences an individual's cognition and perception of the world around them. For example, sociocentric or egocentric values (ie if the individual's identity is collective where they see themselves as part of a kinship or themselves as individualistic) will determine who is approached first when seeking help. This is also linked with cultural identity, eg an egocentric individual may see relationships at an individualistic level and may choose to ignore social expectations and reject arranged marriage whereas a sociocentric individual may follow the norm without any problems.

- **Racism**. Experiences of individual racism and perceived or real institutional racism will also influence where and how help is sought. It will also determine the understanding of the experience of illness and acceptance of treatment. It is likely that past experiences related to racism will impinge on individuals and their carers. It would help to be up-front and honest about it and ask the patient and their carers directly if they have been exposed to racist threats or hassles which may have contributed to their distress.

- **Idioms of distress**. Different cultures use different idioms to express the same type of experience. For example, in Britain, 'I am gutted' will be used to express symptoms of depression and among Punjabi women, 'my heart is sinking' will be seen as an appropriate expression of distress which may indicate underlying depression or anxiety.

Assessing symptoms

- Hallucinations and experiences of possession (which may be erroneously diagnosed as passivity or ideas of control) may have **different diagnostic implications** in some cultural groups.

- In assessing mental state **cultural context** must be seen as essential in understanding the significance of these symptoms. The therapeutic encounter will be influenced by a number of factors such as socio-economic and educational status and previous experiences.

- The folk **support systems** of the patients need to be understood.

- In addition, the significance of **life events** may well vary. Some behaviours are culturally sanctioned, eg speaking in tongues, possession states, but the responses of the individuals and their families may well be different.

- It is helpful to ascertain the **'normalcy'** of some behaviours in certain cultures by asking the carers and/or community leaders to identify the deviancy of certain behaviours.

Using the right language

It is important to understand the role of not only verbal but also non-verbal communication.

- In bilingual patients different psychopathological phenomena may be identified if the patient is interviewed in a secondary language rather than their primary language. The patients may control expression of thought disorder in their secondary language.
- When interpreters are needed, trained professionals should be used. Family members, especially children, should not be used unless there is absolutely no alternative.
- In addition communication with individuals from other cultures may be influenced by cultural norms and nuances, eg close interpersonal distance may be the norm in some cultures but may be seen as threatening in others.
- Ask the interpreter beforehand for useful hints. It may be helpful to learn a few phrases like 'thank you', 'hello' and 'goodbye' which will show the patient your willingness and openness to experiences.

Assessing cultural identity

The cultural identity of any individual will influence the degree of comfort they experience in the society. The main components of cultural identity that clinicians should look out for are:

- religion (practice, frequency, rituals, taboos)
- languages
- attitudes towards relationships, marriage, gender roles, cohabiting etc
- degree of comfort in their own culture and the majority culture
- leisure interests
- dietary habits
- concepts of the self.

These are illustrated below.

Explanatory models

It is good clinical practice that the 'explanatory models' held by all patients to explain mental ill health are assessed. The key questions are:

1 *'What do you think is wrong with you?'*
2 *'What do you think caused it?'*
3 *'What do you think is needed in terms of treatment?'*
4 *'What do you think the outcome is likely to be?'*

These are not dissimilar to checking insight but provide an insight into experiences and suggest a willingness on the part of the clinician to be open in their approach. However, those individuals who come from sociocentric (see above) societies are more likely to hold magico-religious or supernatural explanations and the clinician needs to explore these further.

It must be emphasised that cultures change and individuals assimilate and acculturate. Thus second-generation patients may hold different views from those of their parents and carers. The clinician must be aware of cultural conflict and the impact of migration on individuals as well as the likelihood that patients may be using indigenous or folk models and methods of treatment.

The assessment of black and ethnic minority patients is not difficult if the clinicians are open-minded and willing to explore cultural matters and learn from the patients and their carers.

Summary

- Explore linguistic skills and competency.

- Explore culture, strengths and weaknesses.

- Explore acculturation (eg how comfortable the patients are in the new culture and how much they have given up of their own culture), racism and explanatory models (see above).

- Be aware of your strengths and weaknesses (including prejudices).

- Explore role of family and community.

- Assess
  - symptoms and behaviour in cultural context
  - significance of symptoms culturally
  - idioms of distress
  - perceived outcome
  - what is normalcy and what is deviance in this culture
  - perceived/expected course of illness
  - perceived/expected role of treatment
  - impact of racism
  - cultural identity and world view
  - alternative models of care.

SECTION E

Special Topics

26 Extending your cognitive examination

Why assess cognition?

Cognitive examination can establish:

1 the presence of cognitive disorders

2 the severity of cognitive impairment, which can give an indication as to the severity of the underlying cause (see below)

3 the response to treatment (eg with anti-dementia drugs)

4 important factors in medico-legal cases, ie to inform (not to determine) whether or not someone has the capacity to eg drive a car, make a will, etc.

When to assess cognition

Cognitive assessments cannot take place in isolation from a careful history, especially from an informant. Detailed cognitive assessment is not needed unless:

1 the patient is at high risk through age (risk increasing with age), illness (especially any condition affecting the central nervous system)

2 there is a decline in previously good functioning in the absence of obvious physical or mental illness

3 there is known cognitive impairment and one needs to assess the extent to which different cognitive domains are involved to determine diagnosis, severity and extent of disability.

This section is intended for anyone who is interested in testing other than the basic tests and other cognitive domains. You should also refer to the 3MS in Appendix 5 on page 161 which is a test appropriate for dementia screening in older people.

Praxis

Ask the patient to copy a five-pointed star, two interlocking pentagons and a cube. Dyspraxic patients will not be able to copy these and some surprisingly inaccurate figures can be drawn. These tests may also be supplemented by asking the patient to mimic the use of a comb, pen, or key.

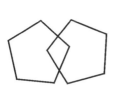

Language

Spontaneous speech

Notice any problems with speaking (not with actually producing speech, which is dysarthria and is a neurological problem). For example circumlocutions are 'the thing you write on paper' paraphasias are 'nearly correct' words, eg wired for radio, substitutions are other words like 'whatsits'.

Naming

The patient is asked to name several things which should start with the commonplace and move to the rare. A good sequence is

Wrist watch ➔ strap ➔ buckle or clasp ➔ winder

Sometimes patients who are dementing will use archaic names like 'wireless' for radio. If they cannot name things, ask them what the items do or how to use them to exclude a visual recognition problem. A standardised test (the Graded Naming test) is available to test this properly.

Comprehension

1 Take out three everyday objects from your pocket like a coin, key and pen.

2 Ask the patient to point to each in turn (single word comprehension).

3 Then ask a series of questions (two- and three-stage comprehension) such as:

> A   put the pen next to the keys
>
> B   pick up the pen after touching the key
>
> C   put the pen between the key and watch and then give me the key.

Repetition

Ask the patient to repeat single words and then phrases and then sentences, eg

1 *'blue / heart / cheese'*

2 *'save the whales / no ifs, ands, or buts'*

3 *'the police arrest the burglars after a chase / tell my friend to bring back the book he borrowed.'*

Reading

Write down a simple command in large letters and ask the patient to read it and do what is said, eg

- *'close your eyes'*
- *'raise your right hand'.*

Spontaneous writing

Ask the patient to write a short sentence.

This screens for dysgraphia. This should not be a signature or a well-known phrase but something made up. If the patient is unsure what to write ask them to write down how they got here or what their favourite television show is.

Executive (frontal lobe) domains

The 'executive' or 'frontal lobe functions' are a broad group of interlinked activities which are very important in psychiatry but are not routinely tested. The functions subsumed under this domain include abstraction (the capacity to appreciate abstract concepts), set shifting (the ability to stop one action or train of thought and to start another), initiation (mental agility). Various tests can be performed.

Initiation

In the absence of nominal dysphasia (see above) verbal fluency tests are good tests of frontal function. You can also pick up perseveration (variations or even the same words generated) or poor short-term memory (forgetting instructions).

- **Categories**. Ask the patient to tell you the names of as many different animals as possible. Do not allow variations of the same animal (eg sheep, lamb). For younger patients 15–20 words are normal; 10 indicates impairment although scores drop with age.

- **FAS test**. If you have time, ask the patient to tell you as many different words beginning with the letters F, A and S as possible in one minute. Normal subjects should produce 15 words for each letter and a total of 30 or fewer words for all three is abnormal. Proper names (eg Fred) or variations of the same word (eg flowered, flowery, floral) are not allowed. This is better than the categories test but takes more time.

Abstraction

- **Similarities test**. Ask the patient what similarities there are between two related items, eg apple and banana, chair and table, shirt and dress. This tests conceptualisation (a frontal lobe function). People with frontal lobe problems would make very concrete interpretations and continue to do so despite being asked to think of other ways in which the two items are alike or different.

- **Cognitive estimates test**. Patients are asked a series of questions which can be answered from general knowledge and reasoning, eg what is the best paid job in the country, how old is the oldest person in the country, what is the population of Britain? Patients with frontal lobe dysfunction will give bizarre or wildly inaccurate answers. The standard test contains 15 questions and should be referred to but a rough idea can be obtained by asking a few questions.

Set shifting and response inhibition

Inhibition of a certain response and shifting to another can be investigated using several tests.

- **Pyramid and square test**

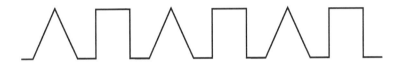

  Ask the patient to continue drawing this sequence of pyramids and squares drawn on one baseline. Only a grossly impaired patient will keep drawing (perseveration) only one of the shapes, usually two or three times. However, it is a quick and easy test to do and interpret.

- **Go – no-go test**

  Ask the patient to raise one finger if you tap under the table twice and two if you tap the table with your finger once. Try it a few times and then try a random series of taps. Patients with frontal lobe deficits cannot inhibit the previous response and will continue raising their finger as in the previous response (perseveration). Like the pyramid and square test this is relatively crude.

The clock drawing test

This is a useful quick and easy screening test which tests frontal (executive) and parietal (praxis) functioning and gives an indication of both the presence and severity of dementia. It is a useful adjunct to the MMSE.

Ask the patient to:

1 *'Draw a large clock face with the numbers put in and then I will tell you what time to put the hands at.'*
2 *'Put the hands to show the time to be ten minutes past five.'*

There are specific ways of scoring this test but at this level all you need to do is to note whether the numbers are correctly placed and sequenced and whether or not the hands are put at the correct time. Sometimes the patient will put the minute hand on the 10 o'clock position, suggesting that 10 is put down first because there is a problem with response inhibition. This sign is known as 'frontal pull'.

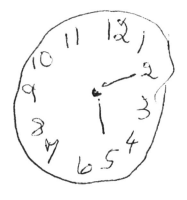

Normal clock

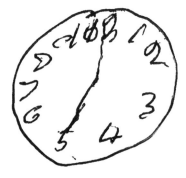

Frontal pull

27 Presenting the case

Style

It is important to put your audience at ease. If you are not at ease yourself this will be difficult so adopt a relaxed (but not too nonchalant) body posture, maintain good eye contact.

Use a conversational style and aim to have the conventional headings of your history flow naturally, eg *'His family is composed of..... There is no family history of psychiatric illness. Now, turning to details of his personal history, he was born...'*

- Speak clearly at a normal conversational rate and do not repeat yourself.

- Do not apologise for any part of your history which seems weak. It may not be so and in any case it makes it seem that you were incompetent rather than that the patient was difficult or unco-operative.

- Correct and consistent use of psychiatric terms is essential. You must be able to define the more common terms on demand, or you might be asked to justify your use of a term, like delusion for example, for the case you are presenting.

- Keep to the allocated time for your presentation.

Content

Whatever the setting (ward round, examination), a good history and examination of the mental state is an important baseline for presentation. However, many students fail to appreciate that the discussion around the case, in terms of differential diagnosis, aetiology, investigation and treatment, are just as important. It makes sense therefore, especially in the setting of a clinical exam, not to devote all your time to taking a history and leave these other issues to chance.

The long case

Introduction

Start by introducing your patient with a one- or two-sentence summary, eg *'I would like to present the case of Mr Brown, a 28-year-old, unemployed, single man admitted informally with ideas of persecution.'*

Presenting complaint

Repeat verbatim what the patient thinks the problem is.

History of the presenting complaint, family history, personal history, MSE, cognitive state

Mention the nature and circumstances of the presenting problems briefly and in the sequence they arose. Then follow the suggested sequence of headings. Skim over negative findings unless they have diagnostic implications. Avoid unnecessary detail.

Physical Examination

Mention briefly any positive findings.

The summary

The summary should aim to give a very short résumé of the relevant points of the case with aetiological factors, differential diagnosis, management and prognosis should be considered. Start along the lines of *'So, in summary, we have a 28-year-old single man without a previous psychiatric history presenting with a two-month history of persecutory delusions....'*

The differential diagnosis

It is always a good idea to offer a diagnosis or differential diagnoses by stating that 'On the basis of my interview with the patient...' in case the patient has not told you everything!

Present in order of decreasing probability (ie most likely diagnosis first). Be prepared to justify any diagnoses you offer and remember that if there is only one possible diagnosis then offer that only. Do not be tempted to give diagnoses for which there is no evidence. Use standard diagnostic terms only (look at the ICD-10 or DSM-IV diagnostic classification books for the terms to use). Remember that illnesses often do not fit easily into standard definitions of an illness so use the 'best fit'. It is also reassuring to keep in mind that psychiatric diagnoses can change with time and a provisional diagnosis is no admission of incompetence but a realistic approach.

Keep in mind possible medical causes for the psychiatric symptoms, eg drugs, metabolic or hormonal disorders (see Appendix 3 for more details).

Aetiology

A useful model of illness is the 'biopsychosocial model' which is an unwieldy way of saying that medical illnesses, personality and environment all interact to produce the illness which is presenting to you. Although best developed in psychiatry this model applies to all branches of medicine (eg it is just as relevant in heart disease or arthritis). The longitudinal view of illness is also important in understanding why the problem is presenting in this particular way and at this particular time. Use the following grid to think about the possible causes

	Biological	Psychological	Social
Predisposing (what made this problem likely)			
Precipitating (why did it start then and not before)			
Perpetuating (why is it still going on)			

Do not feel you have to have something to say for each of the boxes in the grid. It is sufficient just to have thought about it. However, this grid not only helps you understand your patient better but it gives you a better handle on management and makes for a much more impressive presentation!

Management

Investigations

These are 'investigations' in the broadest sense. Do not restrict yourself to a narrow 'medical' concept and the following types of investigation are all possible wherever appropriate.

- **Collateral history**. From relatives and other informants (eg GP), past notes.
- **Physical**. For example, blood tests, chest X-ray, computed tomography scan.
- **Psychological**. For example, neuropsychological tests.
- **Social**. Direct assessment of family situation or residence.
- **Observational**. Further observation over time, eg by nurses on the ward.
- **Occupational**. Assessment by occupational therapists, eg of daily living skills.

Treatment

Be prepared to discuss immediate and long-term treatment plans (use biological, psychological, social headings). Management in psychiatry is multi-disciplinary and integrated so it is important to incorporate this approach in any discussion of management. The psychiatric team usually consists of the doctors, the community and ward-based psychiatric nurses, psychologists, occupational therapists and social workers. Other medical professionals, such as physiotherapists, may be involved. Management will often mean also involving significant non-professional people and agencies like family and friends, housing associations, employers, advocates and patient groups. A broad approach to treatment is a necessary corollary to a broad approach to understanding the causes of mental health problems.

Prognosis

The patient's short- and long-term prospects will be an educated guess and it is important to shape the team's and the patient's expectations of improvement as realistically as possible. Be prepared to provide evidence for the prognosis you offer.

SECTION F

Appendices

Appendix 1:
Psychiatric history checklist

History

Patient details

1 name, age, sex, employment, housing status, marital status and status under Mental Health Act

2 referred by who, why, when admitted?

Presenting complaints

Record each problem briefly in the patient's own words.

History of presenting complaint

Clarify each problem in turn:

1 When did the problem start?

2 What effect does it have on day-to-day functioning?

3 How did it develop?

4 Has any help been sought for it?

5 Are there any associated symptoms?

6 What helps it and what makes it worse?

Screen for symptoms of depression and suicidality, anxiety, changes in thought or unusual perceptions and other recent strange experiences.

Past psychiatric history

Record details of past problems, including hospitalisations and treatments, self harm and detention under the Mental Health Act.

Past medical history

List major illnesses accidents or operations, any current treatments, allergies to prescribed medication.

Personal background

1 Family history. For each member of the family ask about age (or age at death), health, employment, psychiatric history, and relationship with patient.

2 Personal history.

- childhood – birth, developmental milestones, happy childhood, any abuse
- school – formal teaching, relationship with teachers and peers, age when left school, any further training or courses, truancy or bullying
- occupations – jobs taken, for how long, why left, and how long unemployed/retired
- relationships – current and past relationships, how long, why ended/widowed, children
- sexual history – puberty, sexual orientation, first sexual experience, sexual difficulties.

Habits and dependency

Tobacco, alcohol, illicit drugs: quantity, pattern of use, effects.

Forensic history

Record all offences whether convicted or not – especially violent, sexual crimes, or persistent offending, and details of pending cases.

Present social situation

Record details of housing, social support (formal and informal helping networks), daily activities (describe a typical day), finances (debts or allowances).

Personality

Record attitudes to others in social, family and sexual relationships; attitudes to self; predominant mood; leisure activities and interests; reaction pattern to stress.

Appendix 2:
The Mental State Examination (MSE)

Appearance and behaviour

- *Appearance* – level of consciousness, general impression, face, dress.
- *Behaviour* – motor abnormalities and attitude to interview and to yourself.

Speech

- *Production* – spontaneity, speed, volume.
- *Form* – unusual words or sentences.
- Content.

Mood and affect

- *Affect* (observed) – anxious, sad, angry, happy, detached, appropriate, congrous.
- *Mood* (reported) – depression, hypomania, anxiety, irritability.

Thought

- *Delusional content* – persecution, reference, control, jealousy, grandiose, guilt, worthlessness, nihilistic, infestation, amorous, hypochondriacal.
- *Non-delusional content* – phobias, obsessional symptoms.
- *Form* – abnormal fluency (circumstantiality), flow (thought blocking, perseveration, derailment, tangentiality).

Perceptions

- *Illusions.*
- *Pseudo-hallucinations.*
- *Hallucinations* (record modality – auditory, visual, tactile, olfactory, gustatory).
- Depersonalisation.
- Derealisation.

Cognitive state

Minimum of alertness, orientation, attention and concentration, and memory

- *Alertness* – is the patient alert or drowsy?
- *Orientation* – ask name, check time and date, ask where they are or their address
- *Delayed recall* (or long-term memory) – give standard address to remember
- *Attention and concentration* – reverse days of the week
- *Immediate recall* (short-term memory) – read the following numbers slowly and ask the patient to repeat the sequence forwards (as read out) and then backwards. Note the longest correct number of correct sequence forwards and backwards. You can use the following random numbers or make up your own:

6 – 4

8 – 7 – 1

9 – 6 – 3 – 2

0 – 2 – 5 – 0 – 8

7 – 9 – 4 – 1 – 0 – 3

1 – 7 – 0 – 6 – 6 – 9 – 4

Use more formal tests if any deficit is detected in older people.

Insight

- Is the patient aware that there is anything wrong?
- Is the problem within the patient or external?
- If there is anything wrong, does the patient think it is the result of an illness?
- If it is an illness, is it physical or psychological?
- If psychological, can it be helped?
- Is the patient willing to accept help?

Appendix 3: Psychiatric symptoms of physical disorders

This table is not comprehensive and readers are advised to consult standard texts

Physical disorder	Some clinical symptoms/signs	Psychological symptoms
Chronic alcohol misuse	palmar erythema, clubbing, spider-naevi, tremor, gynaecomastia loss of axillary hair	depression, delirium tremens, alcoholic hallucinosis, anxiety, suicidality
Hypothyroidism	weight gain, coarse facies, hair loss, deep voice	depression, dementia
Hyperthyroidism	proptosis, tremor, resting tachycardia	mania, depression, anxiety, psychosis
Addison's disease	tanned, hypotensive	depression
Cushing syndrome	obese, abdominal striae, moon face, hirsutism	depression, mania, psychosis, anxiety
Phaeochromocytoma	episodic hypertension	anxiety
Acute porphyria	episodic abdominal pain, constipation, diarrhoea	depression, psychosis, dementia
Acquired immunodeficiency syndrome (AIDS)	recurrent infections, rash, weight loss	dementia, depression, psychosis
Huntington's disease	choreaform movements	dementia, mania, psychosis
Systemic lupus erythematosus	arthralgia, rash	psychosis
Parkinson's disease	tremor, rigidity, bradykinesia	depression, cognitive impairment, anxiety
Multiple sclerosis	episodic focal neurological signs, nystagmus, ataxia, pyramidal signs	anxiety, personality change, depression, dementia
Epilepsy (temporal lobe)	olfactory hallucinations, déjà vu, automatisms	psychosis, anxiety
Stroke	localising neurological signs, weakness, spasticity	depression, psychosis, dementia

Appendix 4:
Common psychiatric symptoms and possible physical causes

This is not meant to be comprehensive but instead is a guide for the more common physical causes of common psychiatric symptoms.

Psychiatric symptom	Possible physical causes
Depression	hypothyroidism
	cushing syndrome (especially with endogenous steroids)
	parkinson's disease
	stroke
	alcohol
	cancer
Anxiety	hyperthyroidism
	phaeochromocytoma
	epilepsy
	alcohol
Elation	frontal lobe tumours
	multiple sclerosis
	cushing syndrome
Psychosis	epilepsy
	stroke
	alcohol
	hypothyroidism
	porphyria

Appendix 5:
The Modified Mini Mental State Examination (3MS)

This test is a well known screening instrument for dementia which incorporates the original Mini-Mental State Examination (MMSE) and extends it to make it more sensitive in milder forms of memory problems. It is quick to administer, easy to learn, and is fairly reliable and consistent in its results. A form suitable for photocopying and use is to be found on page 166.

Before starting

The test is pretty meaningless without knowing the patient so this could either be a test for a patient who is already known to you or it could be done at a late stage of an initial interview once the presenting complaints are known and cognitive impairment is suspected. Note down any drowsiness, poor eyesight, hearing or any physical impairment of the hands which would impair the patient writing or drawing.

Before starting consider which test you will need to do. If you are pressed for time ask the MMSE questions only. If you have more time the 3MS does not take much more time but your test will be more sensitive. You will need to have with you a score sheet, a pen (or pencil) a spare sheet of paper and a watch.

Introducing the test

Patients might find the test intrusive, frightening or threatening. Introducing the test properly is important since scared, angry or uncooperative people will not do well no matter how intact their cognitive state is. If the presenting problem is their memory then at the beginning mention that you will want to do a test later. If memory problems are accepted by the patient then doing the memory test should not be a problem. If they are not too happy to do a memory test or do not accept that they have a memory problem then saying that this is a quick routine test done on everyone should make them less anxious. If resistance to a memory test is very marked it may be that the patient is trying to avoid showing up cognitive difficulties.

Administering the test

If there are any informants ask them not to prompt unless you ask them to do so. Once the tests starts try to be as non-threatening and conversational as possible. Praise attempts to answer and even when answers are wrong or are missed reassure by saying things like *'well done' 'that's almost right'* or *'don't worry'*. Some people with some insight into their cognitive impairment may become quite angry or anxious as a result of not being able to answer questions. This is known as a 'catastrophic reaction' and when it happens it could be partly the fault of the examiner for not having introduced the test properly.

Scoring and reporting

As this is a formal test battery consistency in scoring is important so 'almost right' answers are noted but not scored. The 3MS cut off score is 77/100 and the MMSE cut off score is 24/30. any interpretation of the score should take into account age and level of education. After doing a test you should report back the results to the patient in a noncommital way eg *'your tests do indicate some problems with your memory. This is because the test is not a definitive assessment of cognitive state nor is it an indicator of likely diagnosis.'* Cognitive assessment scores can be affected by poor attention and concentration from any cause (anxiety, irritability, depression, drowsiness, etc).

When reporting back the 3MS or MMSE to your senior colleagues or examiners do not merely state the score but mention where points have been dropped. For example a score of 25/30 could mean for example one point dropped in five sub-tests or five points in one sub-test. These tests are poorly correlated to any particular region of the brain so do not be tempted to try.

Sub-tests

Practical instructions on the 3MS test administration are given in the test sheet. These points supplement these instructions.

- **Date and place of birth.** This tests orientation to age and can be introduced by asking the patient to confirm their name, age and date of birth as if you are confirming their identity. Make sure you have a reliable independent record of this from another source as otherwise you will have to take their word for it. This is not a test in the MMSE.

- **Immediate recall.** (registration) Make sure that you speak clearly and slowly with a short pause between each word. If the patient is hard of hearing be prepared to speak a little bit more loudly and facing the patient directly. If re-testing use one of the alternative sequences of words.

- **Attention and concentration.** Counting forwards from 1 to 5 is highly learnt information which is retained even in moderate stages of dementia. It is designed to make the patient confident and is not marked. Counting backwards from 5 to 1 is more difficult. A similar approach is taken with the spelling of 'World' with the normal spelling really designed to put the patient at ease (and you are allowed to correct their spelling). If you ask some cognitively impaired patients to spell a word in reverse you might note that they might say that word when trying to recall the three words later.

- **First recall.** The MMSE does not allow 'cued' recall so just ask the patient if they can remember the words. With the 3MS there are two levels of 'cues' - one is a semantic cue which helps the patient guess the word from the meaning, and the other level (which is marked less) gives a list of words and asks the patient to remember which one of these was the word they had to remember. Confabulation is picked up by this test as people who forget can sometimes guess wildly.

- **Orientation to time.** First ask what the date is and you may then get several of the sub-questions answered in this section. If this is not answered try and ask the sequence of questions as shown i.e. from easiest to the most difficult so that people feel confident. Again the MMSE expects a correct answer and the 3MS gives different marks depending on how 'off the mark' the answer is.

- **Orientation to place.** This is straightforward. Remember however that if seeing someone in their home this will be highly learnt knowledge and so present even in severely impaired people. Conversely, if someone is seen in a new place (eg after a recent admission to hospital or at their first visit to a clinic) they may not have much of an idea where they are even though they are cognitively intact.

- **Naming.** In the MMSE this is not very sensitive test and the 3MS sensibly extends it by this bit by asking to name bits of the body. Note any word substitutions (eg *'the thing you write with', 'the bit you shave'*) which suggests more subtle forms of word finding difficulties.

- **Word lists.** You should introduce this by saying that you would like them to generate a list of words and give an example by briefly listing names of cars or foods that you can buy in a supermarket. Then say that you would like them to generate a list of four legged animals in 30 seconds. Note down instances where the number of words generated is very small and any intrusions (ie names from the example lists) or category mistakes (ie naming two legged animals instead). This is a test of executive (frontal) functioning.

- **Abstract thinking (similarities).**This test of abstract thinking is another frontal (executive) test. Record the answers given so that comparisons can be made when re-testing later.

- **Repetition.** Difficulties with patient's hearing and speech production or the examiner's pronunciation may affect this. The 'ands' is so often dropped with a British population that it might be considered as normal.

- **Reading and comprehension.** This again is a simple test of reading but it is the ability to obey the initial instructions more than the reading itself which may affect response. If the patient does not know what to do ask him what it means and then ask *'can you do that?'* Some people with cognitive impairment will be able to read individual letters but not words

- **Writing.** Poor spelling should not be marked against but should be noted in anyone who had a previously good education or job which involved writing

- **Copying and drawing.** The test is a bit more difficult to do than the rest and is therefore fairly sensitive to early problems even if the total score is normal. This is fairly straightforward to score in MMSE. In the 3MS test however you need to score the enclosed figures separately and score the intersection. An early sign of dyspraxia is that one pentagon is correct but the second one is drawn as a square. Other people will only draw one pentagon and you can prompt by asking *'have you copied it exactly as you see it?'*

- **Three stage command.** Make sure the person has heard you correctly and tell them that you will not be repeating the instructions. Make sure they do not have any problem in using any hand. This task picks up problems with attention and concentration, short term memory and hemiagnosia (neglect of one side or another). Keep the paper to the midline of the person and do not hand it to them. Do not mime or demonstrate the actions before the test and do not prompt them during the test in any way. It is difficult not to be helpful to patients who look at you and ask eg *'do I put it on the floor?'*. The best approach is to suppress your helpful nod, keep a fixed smile and adopt a *'whatever you think follows next'* response.

- **Long term memory.** This is the most sensitive test of memory in the 3MS test and is tested without having warned the patient beforehand about five minutes after you had first said the words. Score as in the first recall sub-test above.

The Modified Mini Mental State Examination (3MS) [i]

Patient: _____ Date: _____ Examiner: _____

	3MS score (max score)	MMSE score (max score)

Date and place of birth

I'd like you to tell me the date you where born and where ?
(Score 1 point for each correct answer)

When born?	Year ?		Month ?		Date ?		(3)	
Where born ?	City or Town ?			County ?			(2)	

Registration

I am going to say three words. After I have finished saying all three, I want you to repeat them after me. I want you to remember them because I want you to name them again in one minute.
(Name the following objects, taking at least one second to say each clearly with a pause between each word
Score one point for each one the patient correctly repeats on the first attempt. Repeat up to 5 times only and note number of attempts separately)
Alternatives in case of a repeat test are **shoes, black, , and socks, blue and charity**

Shirt		Brown		Honesty		(3)	(3)
						(2)	

Mental reversal

Can you count from 1 to 5 ?
Coach up to 2 times if needed, if still cannot do it score 0 and do not proceed to next question
Can you now count backwards from 5 to 1 ?
Score 2 if correct, 1 if 1 mistake or 0 if 2 or more mistakes are made

Do you know how to spell the word WORLD ?		(5)	(5)

Ask them to spell the world. Coach them up to 2 times needed. if cannot do it even with assistance score 0 and do not proceed to next question
Can you now spell it backwards ?
Record the reverse spelling below and tick 1 point for each letter in the correct order
D-L-R-O-W

	(9)	(3)

First Recall

Can you remember the three words I asked you to remember a minute ago ?
MMSE Score: give 1 point for each correct word spontaneously recalled
3MS Score: for each word give 3 if spontaneous recall, 2 if cued, 1 if chooses correctly from a list of words and 0 if incorrect even from a list of words

Shirt	3	Brown	3	Honesty	3		
Something to wear ?	2	A colour ?	2	A good personal quality ?	2		
Shoes, shirt, socks	1	Blue, black, brown	1	Honesty, charity, modesty	1		
						(15)	(5)

Orientation to time

MMSE Score: give 1 point for a correct date
3MS Score: score separately as indicated below depending on the answer

What year is it ?		What season is it ?		What month is it ?	
Correct Year	8	Correct Season	2	Correct month (± 5 days)	2
Missed by 1 year	4	Missed by 1 month	1	Missed by 1 month	1
Missed by 2-5 years	2	Missed by >1 month	0	Missed by > 1 month	0
Missed by >5 years	0				
What date is it ?				What day of the week ?	
Correct	3	Missed by 3-5 days	1	Correct	1
Missed by 1or 2 days	2	Missed by > 5 days	0	Incorrect	0

Orientation to place

Give 1 point for each correct answer. 3MS scores 2 points for identifying country or state and MMSE asks for what floor you are on

Where are we now ?	1	(1)	(1)
(this is the only question asked in MMSE, if patient does not know ask the supplementary question only for 3MS)			
Are we in a hospital, office or at home ?			
What floor are we on ?	1		(1)
What city is this ?	1	(1)	(1)
What county are we in ?	1	(1)	(1)
What country (or state) are we in ? *(for 3MS this scores as 2 points)*	1 or 2	(2)	(1)

166

Naming

What do you call this ? *(Show each item names, give 3 seconds to identify score 1 point for each)*

MMSE		3MS		(5)	(2)
Pencil	Watch	Forehead	Elbow		
		Chin	Knuckle		
		Shoulder			

Word finding

How many four legged animals can you name in 30 seconds ?

Score 1 point for each correct answer up to 10 . if no reply by 10 seconds repeat the question. Correct any incorrect answers once only during the test (i.e. not for every incorrect answer)

				(10)	
				(6)	

Similarities

I am going to ask you to tell me in what ways the following are similar-
for example an apple and an orange are similar because they are fruit

(if the first answer is incorrect score it as such but you can tell them the correct answer)

Arm and Leg		Laughing and crying		Eating and Sleeping	
Body parts or limbs	2	Emotions	2	Essential for life	2
Other correct answer	1	Other correct answer	1	Other correct answer	1
Incorrect	0	Incorrect	0	Incorrect	1

Repetition

Repeat what I say. Speak slowly and clearly.

		(5)	
I would like to go out *(2 points if correct, 1 point if 1 or 2 words are missed out)*			
No ifs ands or buts *(for 3MS score 1 point each for 'ifs', 'ands' or 'buts'; for MMSE score 1 point only but subjects in UK can miss out 'ands')*			(1)

Reading and comprehension

Can you read this and do what it says ? *Allow 5 seconds for a response. If subject reads but notes not respond say* Do what it says

For MMSE score 1 if reads correctly and obeys without prompting

		(3)	(1)
Reads and obeys without prompting	3		
Obeys after prompting	2		
Reads aloud only	1		
Does not read or obey	0		
		(5)	(1)

Writing

Please write down the following sentence on this paper 'I would like to go home'

*Use sheet overleaf . Repeat the sentence word by word if necessary once. Allow 1 minute for response Score 1 point for each word but no score for 'I'
For MMSE allow the patient to spontaneously write a sentence and score a maximum of 1*

		(10)	(1)

Praxis (copying and drawing)

I want you to copy this design as best as you can on this paper.

*Use sheet overleaf. Allow 1 minute for copying. Do not penalise for self corrected errors, minor gaps, tremors or overshoots.
For MMSE score 1 point if each pentagon has 5 sides and 5 clear corners and the overlap forms a diamond
For 3MS score separately for each pentagon and the intersecting figure as follows*

	Pentagon 1	Pentagon 2
For 5 approximately equal sides	4	4
For 5 unequal sides	3	3
For other enclosed figure (e.g. square)	2	2
Intersection of two figures has 4 corners		2
Intersection has fewer than four corners		1
	(3)	(3)

Three stage command

I want you to take this paper with your right hand.
Fold the paper in half with both hands and hand the paper back to me

Do not repeat these instructions once the patient has understood (i.e. allow for poor hearing) or coach by miming the movements. Give paper to midline. If patient is left handed use left hand instead. Do not nod or repeat instructions if asked in the middle of test.

		(9)	

Delayed recall

Can you remember the three words I asked you to remember about 5 minutes ago ?

3MS Score: for each word give 3 if spontaneous recall, 2 if cued, 1 if chooses correctly from a list of words and 0 if incorrect even from a list of words

Shirt	3	Brown	3	Honesty	3
Something to wear ?	2	A colour ?	2	A good personal quality ?	2
Shoes, shirt, socks	1	Blue, black, brown	1	Honesty, charity, modesty	1

				100	30

Patient: _____ Date: _____ Examiner: _____

3MS Sheet to show to patient

Read this and do what it says

CLOSE
YOUR EYES

Copy this figure on this sheet

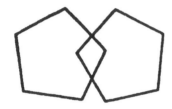

Write sentence here

Appendix 6:
The Alcohol Use Disorders
Identification Test (AUDIT)

A score of 8 in men and 7 in women indicates a strong likelihood of hazardous or harmful alcohol consumption.

1 How often do you have a drink containing alcohol?
(0) Never (1) Monthly or less (2) Two to four times a month
(3) Two or three times a week (4) Four or more times a week

2 How many drinks containing alcohol do you have on a typical day when you are drinking?
(0) 1 or 2 (1) 3 or 4 (2) 5 or 6 (3) 7 to 9 (4) 10 or more

3 How often do you have six or more drinks on one occasion?
(0) Never (1) Less than monthly (2) Monthly (3) Weekly (4) Daily or almost daily

4 How often during the past year have you found that you were not able to stop drinking once you had started?
(0) Never (1) Less than monthly (2) Monthly (3) Weekly (4) Daily or almost daily

5 How often during the past year have you failed to do what was normally expected of you because of drinking?
(0) Never (1) Less than monthly (2) Monthly (3) Weekly (4) Daily or almost daily

6 How often during the past year have you needed a first drink in the morning to get yourself going after a heavy drinking session?
(0) Never (1) Less than monthly (2) Monthly (3) Weekly (4) Daily or almost daily

7 How often during the past year have you had a feeling of guilt or remorse after drinking?
(0) Never (1) Less than monthly (2) Monthly (3) Weekly (4) Daily or almost daily

8 How often during the past year have you been unable to remember what happened the night before because you had been drinking?
(0) Never (1) Less than monthly (2) Monthly (3) Weekly (4) Daily or almost daily

9 Have you or has someone else been injured as a result of your drinking?
(0) No (2) Yes, but not in the past year (4) Yes, during the past year

10 Has a relative or friend or a doctor or other health worker been concerned about your drinking or suggested you cut down?
(0) No (2) Yes, but not in the past year (4) Yes, during the past year

Babor, T.F., de la Fuente, J.R., Saunders, J. and Grant, M. 1992. *AUDIT. The Alcohol Use Disorders Identification Test. Guidelines for use in primary health care.* Geneva, Switzerland, World Health Organisation.

Appendix 7:
Further reading and resources

Recommended supplementary reading:

Hodges, John R, *Cognitive Assessment for Clinicians* (Oxford University Press, 2004)

Sims, Andrew C P, *Symptoms in the Mind: An Introduction to Descriptive Psychopathology (3rd Edition)* (Saunders, 2002)

ICD-10 International Statistical Classification of Diseases and Related Health Problems: Instruction Manual, (World Health Organization, 1992)

Diagnostic and statistical manual of mental disorders: DSM-IV-Tr: Fourth edition, revised (American Psychiatric Publishing Inc, 2000)

Out of Print books:

You may be able to borrow these from your local postgraduate library

Fish, Frank, *Clinical Psychopathology: Signs and Symptoms in Psychiatry,* (J. Wright, 1967)

Leff, Julian, and Isaacs, Anthony, *Psychiatric Examination in Clinical Practices* (Blackwell Scientific Publications, 1978)

Web-site resources:

http://mindmelt.co.uk/trickcyclists/index.htm (look particularly at the section on psychopathology

Index

PASTEST – DEDICATED TO YOUR SUCCESS

PasTest has been publishing books for medical students and doctors for over 30 years. Our extensive experience means that we are always one step ahead when it comes to knowledge of current trends in undergraduate exams.

We use only the best authors, which enables us to tailor our books to meet your revision needs. We incorporate feedback from candidates to ensure that our books are continually improved.

This commitment to quality ensures that students who buy PasTest books achieve successful exam results.

Delivery to your door

With a busy lifestyle, nobody enjoys walking to the shops for something that may or may not be in stock. Let us take the hassle and deliver direct to your door. We will dispatch your book within 24 hours of receiving your order.

How to Order:

www.pastest.co.uk

To order books safely and securely online, shop at our website.

Telephone: +44 (0)1565 752000 Fax: +44 (0)1565 650264

For priority mail order and have your credit card to hand when you call.

Write to us at:

PasTest Ltd
FREEPOST
Haig Road
Parkgate Industrial Estate
Knutsford
WA16 7BR

PASTEST BOOKS FOR MEDICAL STUDENTS

PasTest are the specialists in study guides and revision courses for medical qualifications. For over 30 years we have been helping doctors to achieve their potential. The PasTest range of books for medical students includes:

EMQs for Medical Students Volume 1   1 901198 65 0
Adam Feather et al

EMQs for Medical Students Volume 2   1 901198 69 3
Adam Feather et al

EMQs for Medical Students Volume 3 Practice Papers
     1 904627 07 2
Adam Feather et al

Total Revision: EMQs for Medical Students   1 904627 22 6
Richard Bellamy, Muzlifah Haniffa

Essential MCQs for Medical Finals, Second edition   1 901198 20 0
Rema Wasan, Delilah Hassanally, Balvinder Wasan

Essential MCQs for Surgical Finals, Second edition   1 901198 15 4
Delilah Hassanally, Rema Singh

Essential MCQs in Clinical Pharmacology   1 901198 32 4
Delilah Hassanally, Rema Singh

Essential MCQs in Obstetrics and Gynaecology   1 901198 34 0
Diana Hamilton-Fairley

OSCEs for Medical Students, Volume 1   1 904627 09 9
Adam Feather, Ramanathan Visvanathan, John SP Lumley

OSCEs for Medical Students, Volume 2   1 904627 10 2
Adam Feather, Ramanathan Visvananthan, John SP Lumley

OSCEs for Medical Students, Volume 3   1 904627 11 0
Adam Feather, Ramanathan Visvananthan, John SP Lumley, Jonathan Round

Medical Finals: Passing the Clinical   **0 906896 43 6**
Christopher Moore, Anne Richardson

Surgical Finals: Passing the Clinical Second Edition **1 901198 77 4**
Gina Kuperberg, John S P Lumley

100 Clinical Cases and OSCEs in Medicine   **1 904627 12 9**
David McCluskey

100 Clinical Cases and OSCEs in Surgery   **1 904627 00 5**
Arnold Hill, Noel Aherne

Essential Skills Practice for OSCEs in Medicine **1 904627 38 2**
David McCluskey

Medical Finals: Structured Answers and Essay Questions
                              0 906896 79 7
Adam Feather, Ramanathan Visvanathan, John SP Lumley

**Surgical Finals: Structured Answers and Essay Questions, Second
Edition**   **1 901198 43 X**
Ramanathan Visvanathan, John SP Lumley

Learning by Lists for Medical Students   **1 901198 30 8**
Stuart McPherson

**The Practical Guide to Medical Ethics and Law for Junior Doctors
and Medical Students**
                              1 901198 76 6
Chloe-Maryse Baxter, Mark Brennan, Yvette Coldicott

Radiology for Medical Students   **1 904627 29 3**
Rema Wasan, Alan Grundy, Richard Beese

Clinical Skills for Medical Students: A Hands-on Guide
                              1 901198 86 3
Ian Bickle, David McCluskey, Barry Kelly